PREVENTION'S BEST™
America's #1 Choice for Healthy Living

NO-FAIL FITNESS TIPS

By the Editors of *Prevention* Health Books

RODALE

ST. MARTIN'S PAPERBACKS

Notice

This book is intended as a reference volume only, not as a medical manual. The information given here is designed to help you make informed decisions about your health. It is not intended as a substitute for any treatment that may have been prescribed by your doctor. If you suspect that you have a medical problem, we urge you to seek competent medical help.

The information in this book is excerpted from *Banish Your Belly, Butt, and Thighs Forever!* (Rodale, 2000), *Fat to Firm at Any Age* (Rodale, 1998), and *Busy Woman's Cookbook* (Rodale, 2000).

Prevention's Best is a trademark and *Prevention* Health Books is a registered trademark of Rodale Inc.

NO-FAIL FITNESS TIPS

© 2002 by Rodale Inc.

Cover Designer: Anne Twomey
Book Designer: Keith Biery

ISBN 0–312–98247–X   paperback

Printed in the United States of America

Rodale/St. Martin's Paperbacks edition published May 2002

St. Martin's Paperbacks are published by St. Martin's Press, 175 Fifth Avenue, New York, NY 10010.

10 9 8 7 6 5 4 3 2

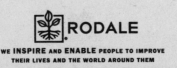

RODALE

WE INSPIRE AND ENABLE PEOPLE TO IMPROVE
THEIR LIVES AND THE WORLD AROUND THEM

Contents

Introduction

If you've squashed your hips into control-top pantyhose, held your breath to zip up your jeans, or struggled into last year's bathing suit, you've experienced firsthand the sobering truth about flab: Left alone, it expands by stunning leaps and bounds. In fact, researchers from the University of Maryland at Baltimore have discovered that unless a woman takes action, her body fat increases by 26 percent with each decade.

No wonder one in three Americans is overweight. Or that two out of three of us feel flabby and long to get fit. Or that we are so desperate to slim down that we spend more than $4 billion a year on weight-loss programs, fat substitutes, and diet drugs. So why does our flab keep on growing? Obesity experts say that we are overlooking the real forces conspiring to make us overweight, forces that you can control.

Our fast-lane lifestyles. Three out of four of us are so busy that we can't find the time for regular physical activity. And the modern conveniences meant to help us save time and effort are actually adding inches to our hips and waists because they keep us sedentary.

Fat-free food. Overindulging in fat-free foods may be the reason that Americans are eating more calories than ever, says nutrition expert John Allred, Ph.D., a biochemist and professor of nutrition in the department of food science and technology at Ohio State University in Columbus. Ironically, despite all the fat-free foods we eat, our *fat* consumption has fallen a mere 6 calories a day, about the amount in one large droplet of corn oil.

Dieting. Yes, dieting can leave you flabby. Low-calorie eating plans encourage your body to burn fewer calories and hoard the body fat you're trying to lose, notes G. Ken Goodrick, Ph.D., assistant professor of medicine at Baylor College of Medicine in Houston. And special weight-loss programs don't give you the skills you need for a lifetime of healthy, satisfying eating.

Eating out. These days we spend about 44 cents of every food dollar eating away from home. With super-size portions and gobs of hidden fat, restaurant meals and takeout food have become a way of life guaranteed to pad hips and thicken waistlines.

Fortunately, you can defeat the forces of flab and get fit by following the no-fail tips in this book. You'll discover a simple, powerful plan that couples good nutrition with fat-burning exercises and toning techniques to help restore your figure. Endorsed by weight-loss experts, these tips don't require you to follow a special diet or a rigid exercise regimen. You simply tailor our program to your likes, your lifestyle, and your budget.

When you mold a healthy eating plan and gentle physical fitness program to suit yourself, you'll stop gaining body fat. You'll enjoy permanent weight loss. You'll feel more energetic and improve your health. And you'll never go hungry or find yourself stuck in an exercise routine that's unpleasant or uncomfortable.

Your weight-loss dream *can* be a reality. All you need do to start on your journey is turn the page.

PART ONE

Fat-Busting Basics

Think Lifestyle Changes, Not Diet

Are you hauling around unwanted pounds? Do you feel as if someone held your body over a copy machine and punched the enlarge button? Stop blaming yourself. Modern life is fattening.

"Our civilization has worked hard to achieve a high standard of living," says obesity expert Richard L. Atkinson, M.D., professor of medicine and nutritional sciences at the University of Wisconsin in Madison and past president of the American Society for Clinical Nutrition. "We enjoy a rich diet. We have labor-saving devices. But we also work long hours and have no time for physical activity. The inevitable consequence is overweight."

When scientists from the National Center for Health Statistics of the Centers for Disease Control and Prevention in Hyattsville, Maryland, weighed a representative sample of Americans, they were startled to discover just how fattening our remote-control lifestyle can be: One in three people was overweight, up from one in four in 1960.

The researchers estimate that from the mid-1970s to the 1990s, the average person gained 8 pounds. Many gained far more. What's more, the pounds-on trend seems to be hitting people earlier than ever. While the number of overweight Americans in their forties has increased somewhat, the proportion of overweight Americans in their thirties went from one in five to one in three. For those in their twenties, overweight doubled from one in ten to one in five.

All told, 32 million of us tip the scales significantly above our ideal body weights.

Experts are quick to blame our sedentary ways for this collective corpulence. "We don't move anymore," says Sue Cummings, R.D., assistant professor at the Institute of Health Professions and a clinical dietitian who specializes in weight loss at Massachusetts General Hospital, both in Boston. "You can even press a button to roll down the car window."

Dead-End Diets

So, in an effort to head off creeping weight gain, we diet. Liquid meals. Public weigh-ins. Prepackaged "diet cuisine." Super-low-calorie regimens. While we desperately want these weight-loss systems to work, the truth is they don't.

"Ninety-five percent of the people who lose weight regain it all within 5 years," says Cummings. And despite the bounty of low-fat, fat-free, and diet foods crowding supermarket shelves, the long-term prospects aren't any better.

Nutrition researchers suspect that those new low-fat and nonfat foods may actually make us fatter in the first place, says John Allred, Ph.D., a biochemist and professor of nutrition in the department of food science and technology at Ohio State University in Columbus and author of Taking the Fear Out of Eating. Overindulging in "guilt-free" goodies, he says, may account for the extra calories Americans are now consuming.

"People tend to think that they can eat a lot of these low-fat items, but sweet foods and snack foods still have a lot of calories," he says. "There's no magic in low-fat foods. If you take in more calories than you burn, you'll be fatter."

The New "Thin" Thinking

Happily, the no-fail fitness program described in this book offers a new promise for success. The cornerstone? It's a program you create for yourself. "If a person has power over her food choices and exercise program, then she will be successful in any weight-loss attempt," says Anne Dubner, R.D., a nutrition consultant in Houston and a spokesperson for the American Dietetic Association. "The key is you have to play a part in all the decisions."

The foundation of a healthy weight-loss program proved in studies of women who have successfully lost weight and kept it off, isn't a diet at all. It's a new way of thinking. "It's all about redefining success," says Cummings. "You have to think about your own life and your own body and what's right for you."

Following this program requires creative problem solving. You can melt down modern-day barriers that keep you from achieving a healthy weight by devising a program that flexes with the demands of your unique life, says Susan Kayman, R.D., Dr.P.H., program coordinator of regional health education for the Kaiser-Permanente Medical Group in Oakland, California.

"A woman may have to learn some coping skills to handle what's going on in her life. It's the first and most powerful step," says Dr. Kayman, who has studied women who succeeded in maintaining their goal weight. "Without these skills, you may eat to feel good rather than thinking about and resolving the real issue bothering you. Or you end up watching TV instead of exercising."

Of course, this involves a healthy eating program, but one tailored to your own needs and desires. One that leaves you feeling satisfied, includes your favorite foods, and focuses on nutritious, low-fat meals. One that helps you deal with the weak moments when you're most vulnerable to overeating.

It also includes a fitness plan—the kind you enjoy and have the time to do. And if you must set pound-shedding goals, it calls for small, smart, reasonable steps—such as losing weight in increments of no more than 5 to 10 pounds at a time.

"If you eat healthy food, find time for fitness, and work on problem solving, you can stabilize at a lower weight and improve your health risks a lot," says G. Ken Goodrick, Ph.D., assistant professor of medicine at Baylor

Battling the Nine-to-Five Bulge

"At work, we mostly move our fingers at keyboards and move our mouths, talking. We don't move our bodies," says Abby King, Ph.D., assistant professor of medicine and health research and policy at Stanford University School of Medicine.

Small wonder that one-third of American women are overweight. Thanks to mechanization, many of the little activities that once burned workaday calories have been supplanted by computers, elevators, fax machines, copiers, and answering machines.

"People used to climb stairs more often," notes Ralph Paffenbarger, M.D., Dr.P.H., professor emeritus of epidemiology at Stanford University School of Medicine, who has studied physical activity on the job. "They typed on typewriters and had to press the keys down. If you needed

College of Medicine and associate director of the Behavioral Medicine Research Center, both in Houston. "You'll lower your risk of cardiovascular disease, diabetes, high blood pressure, and some forms of cancer. And you'll have more energy."

Resist the Remote Control

When it comes to fitness, you can maximize healthy weight loss by taking advantage of your body's three-way calorie-burning system. "Sixty percent of the calories you use up are burned by your lean muscles during everyday activities," says Cummings. "Another 30 percent are burned by intense physical activity, and 10 percent are burned during digestion."

a file, you hopped up and went to the filing cabinet. There's been a big shift away from physical activity in our working lives."

The antidote? Create more physical activity at work. "You can make small changes that will help prevent obesity and lower your risk for diseases such as heart disease and diabetes," Dr. King notes. "And these activities also help fight stress."

Her top suggestions: Take the stairs instead of the elevator. Deliver messages in person, not by phone or e-mail. Take a walking break, or even schedule a meeting as a walk.

"If you can work in three 10-minute sessions of exercise a day, it goes a long way toward helping prevent overweight and improving health," she says. "Aim for moderate intensity—the pace of a brisk walk."

Start with something aerobic. Choose an aerobic fitness activity—such as walking, biking, swimming, or aerobic dance—that you can engage in three times a week. "Aerobic exercise mobilizes fat," says Cummings. And it takes just 30 minutes of physical activity to activate that fat-burning power.

Add strength training. With simple weights, you can build more muscle. Using weights will not only burn more calories during exercise but also rev up the rate at which your body burns calories to sustain itself all day, says Cummings.

Get up and around. Get out of your chair at work or your sofa at home, suggests clinical psychologist Abby King, Ph.D., assistant professor of medicine and health research and policy at the Stanford University School of Medicine. After all, for every flight of stairs you climb, you burn 8 to 10 calories.

See Food in a New Light

Skipping meals and going without food are counterproductive. When 99 normal-weight women revealed their weight-maintenance secrets to researchers at Winthrop University in Rock Hill, South Carolina, the value of regular eating was obvious: These women ate three meals a day—and most added at least one snack. They even indulged in occasional fried foods, desserts, sweet sodas, or rich sauces. So they actually ate a few more calories than women who skipped meals, says researcher Patricia Giblin Wolman, R.D., Ed.D., professor of human nutrition and chairperson of the department of human nutrition at Winthrop University. "But," she adds, "they seemed to burn it off."

Why? "Frequent eating works with your metabolism, which speeds up a little each time you eat," says Dr. Wolman. "Also, if you eat regular meals, you'll be less likely to feel ravenously hungry and overeat at one meal."

What's on the plates of successful weight maintainers? It's not "diet" food. In Dr. Kayman's study, women who kept weight off didn't think of their food choices as temporary weight-loss plans. "While people who regained weight they'd lost tried special diet foods and formulas, maintainers adjusted to a meal plan they could follow all the time." The basic elements follow.

Bring on the fiber. The best plan turns out to be a high-fiber, low-fat eating plan that you can enjoy for a lifetime, says Dr. Goodrick. So choose more fruits, vegetables, and whole grains.

Give fat the slip. Shy away from full-fat dairy products, fat-marbled meats, oils, and fried foods.

Dr. Goodrick advocates slowly reducing the amount of fat in your diet to 30 percent or less of total calories—down from the 37 percent that most people eat. "Your weight slowly falls to a level you can maintain," he says. "It's a no-diet approach."

Leap the Mental Barriers

Your mind is your number-one weight-loss tool. That's what Dr. Kayman discovered when she compared two groups: 30 women who shed pounds and kept them off and 44 others who lost weight and then regained it.

"Maintainers made decisions to lose weight and then solved problems that stood in the way, like stress and time constraints," she says. "They persisted until new ways of eating and exercising were established. If the first thing they tried didn't work for them, they didn't give up."

But when life threw the relapsers a curveball, they responded by overeating and by skipping exercise sessions.

"Both groups of women faced the same kinds of stressful problems," Dr. Kayman says. "The difference was how they dealt with it. Women who put their well-being first got over the problem barriers. They found ways to keep eating healthy food and to keep on exercising. The relapsers didn't."

To overcome your own weight-loss barriers, first identify the real problem, Dr. Kayman suggests. If you overeat at night, the real problem may be that you're overworked and come home feeling stressed-out. "Then you ask yourself, 'Why am I working so hard? How can I change this?'" she says. "You may try talking to your boss, socializing more with coworkers, or delegating more work. The point is that you find solutions that work for you, and you keep experimenting until you find the one that's right for you."

Redefine Success

At Baylor University's Behavioral Medicine Research Center, Dr. Goodrick and other weight-loss experts have identified other themes among people who have stepped off the diet roller coaster and stayed off: These people focused on health rather than appearance, built new levels of self-esteem, and set realistic weight goals.

"The theory we go by is that being happy, having a constructive and meaningful life, and enjoying good relationships are the ultimate goals, and they're things you can have whether or not you're thin," Dr. Goodrick says.

"Success is not a low number on the bathroom scale," says Cummings. "It's about better health and a more fulfilling life. You can significantly improve your health by losing just 10 or 15 pounds. I work with one woman whose weight went from 188 to 170, and she feels great about herself. She's exercising every day and eating well, and even got out of a lousy job because she worked on self-esteem. Work to reach your natural weight, not some fictitious ideal."

Personalize Your Program

Quick weight-loss schemes or rigid eating plans won't take you from fat to firm—or help you stay there. What will? Trusting yourself and meeting your own particular needs—whether it's for an afternoon cookie, a slow-and-easy walking plan, or regular snacks to keep hunger at bay.

"The very idea of a diet is the opposite of what works," says Susan Kayman, R.D., Dr.P.H., program coordinator of regional health education for the Kaiser-Permanente Medical Group in Oakland, California, who has studied women who successfully shed excess weight. "What really helps women lose weight and keep it off is very individual solutions."

Dr. Kayman found that women who had maintained a new, lower body weight designed their own plans. Each had her own personal strategy that fit her life, her schedule, and her tastes, she notes.

When you customize a program to meet your own, unique needs, you'll see steady, positive changes that can last a lifetime, Dr. Kayman says. You'll learn to trust your ability to listen to your body and to firm and nourish it in your own way. More and more experts are convinced that this customized approach is the only route to achieving and maintaining a healthy body weight.

That's exactly what this book can help you accomplish. It's a set of tools you can use to design a custom-tailored firm-up plan that's perfect for you now and in years to come.

The Future You

We'll give you the latest information and practical advice—from leading doctors, nutritionists, psychologists, personal trainers, and even fashion experts—on low-fat eating, fitness, self-esteem, and looking good, with dozens of strategies for customizing the program to meet your own needs.

When you adapt a plan to fit your lifestyle, there's a good chance that you can follow it year after year, notes Anne Dubner, R.D., a nutrition consultant in Houston and a spokesperson for the American Dietetic Association.

"If you want the magic in weight loss, get a mirror," Dubner says. "The person you see in the mirror is the one who will lead you to success."

Here's how you can achieve and maintain a healthy weight—by doing it your way.

Goal #1: Lose Body Fat

The "twin engines" of fat burning—easy aerobic workouts and healthy, low-fat eating—are the best ways to reduce body fat, says I-Min Lee, M.D., Sc.D., assistant professor of medicine at Harvard Medical School.

What to do. Choose a workout you love—whether it's walking, swimming, pedaling an exercise bike in your bedroom, or jogging around the park. Follow a satisfying lowfat, high-fiber eating plan that includes your best-loved foods. Try recipe makeovers for your all-time favorites. And use strategies to help you cope with special situations—like meals away from home, holiday dinners, and cooking for a family that likes high-fat fare.

"Exercise actually does more than burn calories while you're doing it," Dr. Lee says. "It motivates people to stick with a good eating plan. It gives you a psychological edge. If you've just walked 3 miles, you may be less likely to give in to a slice of cake or a candy bar."

Benefits. When you lose body fat, you look sleeker, feel more energetic, and may—if your aerobic-fitness choice is a weight-bearing exercise like walking or aerobic dance—build stronger bones, says Ralph W. Cygan, M.D., clinical professor of medicine and director of the weight-management program at the University of California, Irvine, College of Medicine. You also lower your risk for diabetes, high blood pressure, and heart disease.

Goal #2: Gain Firmer, Trimmer Muscles

A strength-training routine at an easy pace for 1½ hours a week will supercharge your firm-up program without building bulky, muscle-bound arms and legs, says William Evans, Ph.D., professor of applied physiology and nutrition and director of the Noll Physiological Research Center at Pennsylvania State University in University Park and author of *Biomarkers: The 10 Keys to Prolonging Vitality*.

What to do. Choose small barbells and dumbbells, resistance bands that look like rubber bands, or machines like Nautilus.

Benefits. Working with weights creates shapely, toned muscles and more muscle mass that burns more calories 24 hours a day, reversing the metabolic slowdown that can make women fat as they age, Dr. Evans says. Weight training also protects and strengthens bones.

Goal #3: Love What You Eat, Eat What You Love

Forget about dieting. Instead, reach for three meals a day, plus snacks. There's room for the foods you love—whether it's steak Diane, blue cheese dressing on fresh salad greens, or chocolate chunk ice cream.

What to do. Eat what you like best. "There are no bad foods," notes Dubner. "It's important to keep eating what you really like, or you'll feel deprived. You just have to know how to do it."

Benefits. By incorporating your favorite foods into your eating plan, you get the nutrition you need to maintain strong bones, protect yourself against disease, and stay alert and energetic all day. You also get the tastes and eating experience you enjoy without guilt or second-guessing.

Goal #4: Feel Wonderful—Now

Learn to value yourself more highly and take new steps toward the life you want.

What to do. Customize your plan by identifying traps that keep you from enjoying the body you have.

Benefits. You'll gain freedom from a negative body image, and freedom to get on with your life and do the things you want to do.

You can stop playing the "if only . . ." game, too. By boosting self-esteem, you can feel and look your best right away. No need to say, "If only I were skinny, then I would feel attractive or have a scintillating social life or get a new job." You can do it now.

"You don't have to lose 20 or 30 pounds in order to achieve what you want in life or have good relationships or be creative and constructive," says G. Ken Goodrick, Ph.D., assistant professor of medicine at Baylor College of Medicine and associate director of the Behavioral Medicine Research Center, both in Houston. "You can be happy and enjoy yourself now."

Concentrate on What You *Can* Change

Three women get together for lunch. One of them, a harried woman whose life is filled with young children and a full-time job, orders a turkey sandwich, hold the mayo, and don't forget the dessert menu. The oldest woman, who works part-time when not tending house, asks for the diet plate—fruit salad and cottage cheese. The youngest woman, who is single, active, and loving it, hasn't eaten anything yet today, and she's starving. She orders a taco salad in a shell.

All three of these women think they are on a diet.

We'd like to introduce you to Margie, Sarah, and Ann, three completely different women who have one big thing in common: They want to lose weight.

- Margie, 40, wants to lose 20 pounds from her hips and backside, which is the extra weight that she has put on since having two children.
- Sarah, 52, is a career dieter. She has 30 pounds to lose—weight that she's lost and regained (plus a little more) over and over again.

16

- And finally there is Ann, 29 and single. She has only 10 pounds to lose, but it's 10 pounds that have settled mostly on her thighs and backside within the last few years.

Margie, Sarah, and Ann are composites, based on what surveys reveal—and weight-loss experts confirm—to be the most common types of women dieters. Margie is the stressed-out career woman who blames her weight gain on having children. Sarah is the nurturing, sedentary, plump mother who spends an inordinate amount of time in the kitchen. Ann is the life-at-full-speed single who hardly thinks about her health. You probably already recognize yourself—or parts of yourself—in one or more of them.

Margie believes that her two pregnancies have left her heavy forever. Sarah believes that menopause—combined with a lifetime of dieting—has ruined her chances of ever being thin again. And Ann believes that her thighs are a genetic inheritance over which she has no control. Are they right?

Well, yes and no. The women's beliefs are, for the most part, half-truths. The whole truth encompasses two realities: Biology plays a role in our size and shape, but we determine how much of a toll it will ultimately take.

"At 20, you usually have the body you were born with, but at 40 or 60, you have a body that reflects the way you lived your life," says Edith Hogan, R.D., a registered dietitian in Washington, D.C., and spokesperson for the American Dietetic Association. "One key to successful weight loss is learning to work with, not against, who you are and what you've been given. Some things you can change, and some you can't."

The Hormone Connection

While calories, fat, and energy expenditure determine to a great extent how much weight you'll gain throughout your life, one other factor figures into the equation—hormones.

Hormones are naturally occurring chemicals that circulate throughout our bodies. Their job is to carry a message from one organ of the body to another, influencing how the second organ will behave. In women, for example, the ovaries secrete estrogen and progesterone, reproductive hormones that play a big role in pregnancy, breast development, and 400 other bodily functions—including fat storage. They also produce the male hormones testosterone and dehydroepiandrosterone (DHEA), albeit in much smaller amounts than men generate.

To a degree, hormones influence our weight and shape. Until recent years, many doctors (and women) assumed that we had little power over our body types, our fat storage, and our life cycles.

That thinking has changed. Research shows that the way we eat, our activity levels, and our ability to handle stress will affect our hormones—and, in turn, our hormones will affect our weight and body shape, says Elizabeth Lee Vliet, M.D., founder and medical director of HER Place women's health centers in Tucson and Dallas. The upshot: You can learn how to help your body handle hormonal changes over the years.

Pregnancy, Cellulite—and Winter

Three things about her weight bug Margie. First, after each of her two pregnancies, she retained 10 extra pounds. Second, she always gains about 7 pounds during the winter, bringing her total close to 30 extra pounds for 6 months of the year. Third, the fat she has accumulated on her hips and thighs isn't attractive; Margie has cellulite, and it keeps her from wearing shorts in the summer, even though she's not quite so heavy then.

Margie assumes that these weight changes are inevitable. She wants to eat well and exercise, but she thinks her particular problems have no solutions. Here's what she needs to know.

Pregnancy. If a woman is at her correct weight when she becomes pregnant, doctors recommend that she gain between 25 and 35 pounds to support and nurture her developing child. Underweight women should gain between 28 and 40 pounds, while overweight women are advised to gain between 15 and 25 pounds. No matter how heavy she is, a woman should never diet while she's pregnant unless she is doing so under the guidance of a doctor or dietitian.

Of 30 pounds gained during pregnancy, for example, only 7 of those pounds are comprised of fat. Amniotic fluid, other tissues, and the baby itself make up the rest and are lost during the birth. So a new mother should have only a few pounds to lose after her baby is born. Women will also notice changes in the shape of their breasts (especially if they breast-feed) and belly, which has stretched to accommodate a full-term child. Likewise, their hips may also widen a bit just before birth. These changes are due not to fat accumulation but to changes in the tissues and bones during pregnancy and lactation.

What you can change: If you retain any more than 4 extra pounds for more than a year or two after giving birth, it's due to your diet and lifestyle, not the pregnancy, says Hogan. Most women should be able to get back to their pre-pregnancy weights, or just a couple of pounds above.

While you can't change the actual shape of your breast tissue, weight training can give your breasts a little more lift by increasing the strength of your pectoral, or chest, muscles. Extra folds of skin can't be exercised off, but losing unwanted fat through diet and exercise can get rid of tummy rolls. Hips that widened to accommodate pregnancy cannot be changed, unless the extra width is from a layer of fat. (If you can pinch it, it's fat.)

Cellulite. Although cellulite looks different from other fat, it really isn't. It looks dimpled because of the way the fat is connected to the muscle underneath—strands of connective tissues pull tight where the fat is thickest (usually on the hips, buttocks, and thighs). Not everyone who has a lot of body fat has cellulite, and some slender women have cellulite. The tendency to develop cellulite seems to have a lot to do with genetics and age, says Dr. Vliet. Women are more prone to cellulite than men.

What you can change: You can certainly change the amount of fat on your body. This book shows you how. And when you reduce the amount of fat, you'll reduce the appearance of cellulite. If, however, you lose excess body fat but what remains is still in the form of cellulite, over-the-counter products and exercise may help to temporarily improve its appearance, says Dr. Vliet. But no over-the-counter cream or beauty salon treatment will actually get rid of cellulite. She adds that the best way to diminish your risk of developing cellulite in the first place is to cut down on processed foods, which tend to be higher in fat and salt, drink fewer sodas, and increase your water intake and exercise.

Winter weight gain. We tend to be less active in winter, says Dr. Vliet. That can prompt weight gain, but hormones also play a part. Less sunlight means that our bodies produce more melatonin, a hormone that regulates our sleep–wake cycles. "Like bears, we 'hibernate' to some degree," Dr. Vliet explains. "But remember, part of the bear's ability to hibernate depends on its ability to store fat, which is helped by melatonin."

Other hormonal influences: decreased levels of both estradiol (a naturally occurring female hormone) and a mood-regulating chemical in the brain called serotonin, Dr. Vliet says. For some women, carbohydrate cravings seem to increase in the winter, and they also contribute to the accumulation of extra winter pounds.

What you can change: Fight the urge to stay indoors, says Dr. Vliet. Instead, get out in the sun and exercise. "Eating high-fiber foods and numerous, smaller meals within a healthy winter diet will also keep your weight closer to that which you enjoy during spring and summer," she adds. High-fiber foods tend to be lower in fat and calories, and eating smaller portions, more often, increases your metabolic rate.

Age, Menopause, and Yo-Yo Dieting

Sarah has spent her lifetime struggling with her weight. Now that she has hit (and passed) the age of 50, the latest changes in her figure are all the more discouraging. With menopause, her body has morphed from a generous hourglass shape into a round apple, and she feels flabbier than ever.

Meanwhile, just the idea of another diet is enough to send her running for the hills. And rightly so. "Sarah's metabolism has most likely slowed down in response to her years of dieting and being inactive," says Blenda Eckert, R.D., a registered dietitian in Clarksville, Maryland. "Another episode of simply cutting down on calories won't help Sarah lose weight anymore."

Does that mean Sarah has to give up? Absolutely not. She just has to do things differently this time. Here's what Sarah and women like her need to consider.

Aging and menopause. At one time, doctors thought there was nothing women (or men) could do to fight the aging process—our bellies got bigger, our muscles went flabby, and everyone ate less but gained more weight.

Now the effects of aging are no longer considered inevitable, says Diana Dell, M.D., assistant professor of obstetrics and gynecology at the Duke University Medical Center in Durham, North Carolina. "The things that really change as you grow older are your muscle mass and activity level, which, in turn, affect your body shape and weight. If you build and maintain muscle and stay active, then your weight won't change very much."

The hormonal changes that accompany menopause do, however, affect a woman's metabolism and, as a result, her weight. "Ovarian hormones, such as estrogen and progesterone, are not just reproductive hormones," says Dr. Vliet. "They also have a metabolic role in the body and help you to build muscle and bone. So when these hormones decline, so do muscle and bone mass, and the body stores more fat."

With the drop in female hormones, the small amounts of adrenal hormones that women (and men) produce come into play, changing that hourglass figure into an apple shape.

Estrogen replacement medications, such as Alora, that supply estradiol can help to prevent muscle and bone loss as well as the weight gain associated with menopause, says Dr. Vliet. Progesterone, on the other hand, promotes weight gain and for various reasons is often combined with estrogen. Estrogen-like compounds found in some plants, such as soy, may contribute to weight distribution and the maintenance of a healthy female body shape.

What you can change: Regardless of whether or not you take some form of hormone replacement therapy, if you overeat and don't exercise, you won't slim down or shape up. If you ask your muscles and bones to move, then they'll stimulate the process of using fat for fuel.

The solution is to do activities that are aerobic (such as walking) and weight-bearing (walking, again, and strength training), says Dr. Vliet. Both moving regularly and building muscle are imperative.

Yo-yo dieting. Repeated weight losses and gains change the structure and number of your fat cells, which can ultimately make it much easier for you to regain weight you've worked hard to lose. Fat cells first increase in size during a weight-gain period, but when they reach their maximum size, they divide, creating two fat cells where once there was one. Once created, fat cells never disappear; they can only shrink.

What you can change: Fat cells will always be able to change size—to grow or shrink—so losing weight is not impossible.

"Focus on your lifetime plan to keep weight off, not just your short-term diet to lose weight quickly," says Michael Steelman, M.D., a weight-loss specialist in Oklahoma City. Experts agree that exercise keeps weight from returning.

PMS, Body Shape, and Heredity

Despite usually staying within 10 pounds of her goal weight, Ann is plagued by a week of PMS every month that adds another few pounds to her frame before menstruation. She feels so bloated and fat that she has accumulated a second wardrobe of "period pants and skirts." A size larger than her regular wardrobe, these clothes help Ann feel more comfortable at a time when she's already prone to crying.

But two other things bother Ann even more than her premenstrual weight gain. She harbors a secret that both embarrasses and frightens her: Her mother is very overweight, more than 100 pounds. So even though she has only 10 pounds to lose now, to Ann they're a sign of what's to come. At this point, she has cellulite on her thighs, and her body is quite pear-shaped. She obsesses about her weight and "heavy thighs" and feels doomed that one day she will follow in her mother's footsteps.

Ann's worries are valid, but her situation isn't hopeless. Here's where she stands.

Premenstrual bloating. Seven to 10 days before their periods begin, most women gain a few pounds because of water retention. Progesterone levels instigate these temporary weight gains, which disappear once periods start. It's a natural part of the reproductive cycle, although not all women experience bloating and other premenstrual symptoms.

What you can change: A few simple changes can reduce the tendency to retain water, says Dr. Vliet. She recommends cutting some salt from your diet, increasing your activity level, eating more fiber, and consuming more magnesium, a mineral that plays a role in fluid balance. If problems persist, Dr. Vliet recommends having your hormone levels checked.

If you've consistently gained an extra pound or two *after* your period, then you've been eating too much before and during your period, not retaining water.

Pears and apples. Although women come in all shapes and sizes, they tend to accumulate fat in two ways—in the shape of a pear or an apple.

"A pear gains weight in her lower body—the hips, thighs, and backside—while an apple gains weight around her abdomen," says Dr. Vliet. "The balance of female versus male hormones determines who becomes a pear and who becomes an apple."

Most women are pears until middle age. "Your body shape changes as you grow older because of the hormonal changes that occur as the years go by," Dr. Vliet explains. "After menopause, we produce less estrogen and progesterone, and that causes us to begin to gain weight the way men do, over the tummy." This is due to the relative excess of testosterone and DHEA as estradiol declines, she says.

Ann believes that all the extra calories from her late-night food fests accumulate on her thighs. The truth is that the first few pounds might head to her lower body, but the rest distribute themselves all over. "Everyone has a particular pattern of weight gain," says Dr. Steelman. "You can't control or change those genes, but no one gains weight in just one place."

What you can change: The best strategy is to not gain weight in the first place. If you've already accumulated a few extra pounds, you can still affect the shape of your lower body with resistance training and abdominal exercises—if you also keep the fat off through diet and exercise, says Rick Kahley, an exercise physiologist and certified personal trainer in Macon, Georgia.

Genetics. If you have two obese parents (meaning that they weigh 20 percent or more than they should), the chance that you will be obese is about 80 percent. If one of your parents is obese, your chance is 23 percent. If neither of your parents is obese, you have less than a 10 percent chance of being obese. Likewise, some families or ethnic groups have a genetic tendency to gain weight or, conversely, have a high basal metabolic rate (the number of calories a person burns at rest).

Two factors seem to be a part of heredity and weight gain. First, scientists have identified a gene (called the obese gene) that is responsible for leptin, a hormone that lets you know that you're full and can stop eating. Researchers believe that in some people this gene doesn't work properly, and their cell receptors don't recognize signals that help them stop eating.

Among relatively few women, the second possible factor is adaptation. Until this century, food wasn't plentiful for most human beings. So historically, our bodies have learned to store what they get to make sure they still have energy available during times when food is scarce. Over the course of several generations, some ethnic groups—Pima Indians, in particular—have become more adept than others at storing food as fat, in order to protect against times of famine, says Dr. Vliet.

What you can change: It takes work to fight your genes, but it can be done. "If Ann commits herself to staying in good physical shape, then she won't gain the fat that she's afraid of," says Grace Mello, R.D., a registered dietitian in Westerly, Rhode Island. "Ann and her sisters and parents may share the same basic shape. But if one works out regularly and eats well and the others don't, you will see a difference in their figures."

Biology Is Not Destiny

Yes, hormones and our genetic backgrounds do influence your size and shape. You can't change your height, your sex, or the basic physics of your body, but you have a lot of control over your weight.

"People who have been successful at weight loss tend to have a positive outlook about their food intake and exercise habits, weigh themselves about three times a week, exercise consistently, and keep a record of what they eat and their activity," says Eckert.

Why do these things work? Because many overweight people don't accurately judge how much they eat against how little they exercise. "Behavior and habits are really the deciding factors for most people regarding weight," says Hogan. "The eating, exercise, and attitude habits you practice throughout your life have much more of an impact on your weight than genetics."

PART TWO

The Fat-Burning Diet

10 Keys to Eating Lean

Stop treating food as the enemy! You can't live without it, so you might as well make peace with it. And the sooner you accept that no foods are inherently bad and that you can enjoy a rich and rewarding relationship with food, the sooner your battle against excess weight will be won.

Of course, barring sudden illness, weight loss doesn't just happen. As with everything else, you need a plan—and a set of guiding principles. Below are 10 that weight-loss experts swear by.

Keep in mind that for results to be permanent, you have to lose weight *your* way. What put your sister, mother, or best friend in size 10 jeans won't necessarily do the trick for you. So mold the following principles into a program that you can actually enjoy—and stick with.

1. Take stock of what you're eating now. The only way you'll really know is to write down what you eat for several days. A food diary is an effective weight-loss tool, says Suellyn Crossley, R.D., a registered dietitian and director of Healthy Weight Management at Florida Hospital Celebration Health in Orlando. She has all of her clients keep one for at least three days.

2. Shop smart. "You have to eat to lose weight!" says Megrette Hammond, R.D., a registered dietitian in Nottingham, New Hampshire, who specializes in eating disorders and motivation issues. The trick is to eat differently than you do now. The easiest way to do that is to become a smart shopper—one who uses simple substitutions to cut calories and grams of fat without missing them.

3. Balance your fat intake. Become aware of the fat in foods so you can learn to balance high-fat items with low-fat ones. Says Toni Bloom, R.D., a registered dietitian in San Jose, California, who counsels people all day long: "There's definitely room in every diet for high-fat foods. But you have to know which foods actually do have more fat so you can plan to eat less of those."

4. Learn the difference between hunger and thirst. "People often think they're hungry when they're actually thirsty," says Christine Palumbo, R.D., a registered dietitian in Naperville, Illinois. She recommends that you drink a glass of cold water when the urge to nibble hits. Then wait to see if your hunger disappears after a few minutes. "Water gives you a sense of fullness," explains Ann S. Litt, R.D., a registered dietitian in Bethesda, Maryland.

5. Fill up on fiber. Logically enough, high-fiber foods are filling. They prevent you from overeating. "Fiber-rich foods take up more space in your stomach, so you feel satisfied longer," says Debra Indorato, R.D., a registered dietitian and the owner and consulting dietitian for Approach Nutrition and Fitness in Allentown, Pennsylvania.

For general health as well as cancer prevention, the National Cancer Institute recommends 20 to 35 grams of fiber a day. Most people are lucky if they get half that, but it's not difficult to work fiber into your diet. Fruits, vegetables, dried beans, cereals, and whole-grain breads have plenty.

6. Eat all day long. Most weight-loss experts agree that eating small meals, more frequently, throughout the day really keeps you satisfied—and prevents a detour to binge city later in the evening. "When people front-load their calories (by eating earlier in the day) and then eat every 3 to 4 hours, they appease their appetites," says Bloom.

7. Stop eating when you're satisfied. Learn to distinguish between fullness and satiety. Fullness is the weight of food in your stomach. "You can feel full from 10 heads of lettuce, but will you be satisfied?" asks Hammond. Probably not, so you just keep on eating.

Satiety is the level of satisfaction you get from eating. And the best way to be satisfied is to eat foods with a variety of flavors, colors, and textures. Forget a cheeseburger and fries, with their similar color and texture. Think instead of chicken parmigiana, baby carrots, fettuccine, and a tossed salad with mixed lettuce and chopped yellow bell peppers.

8. Don't skip meals. It's a sure way to deprive your body of adequate calories for energy, not to mention valuable disease-fighting nutrients and phytochemicals, compounds in fruits and vegetables that can improve your health. Dietitians Crossley and Indorato see skipping breakfast as a major deterrent to successful weight loss.

9. If you want it, eat it—sometimes. "You don't need to deprive yourself while trying to lose weight," Indorato says emphatically. "You can still eat your favorite foods." She actually has her weight-loss clients list all their favorite foods, especially those they absolutely cannot live without. Then she teaches them how to eat smaller portions of these foods and relish each bite.

10. Enjoy what you eat. Many people eat so fast that they don't actually taste the food. And because of that, they aren't really satisfied—which sets them up for overeating later on.

This concept is seconded by dietitian Litt. "I tell my clients to eat something they really like every day because it tastes good, not necessarily because it's good for them."

The 21 Best Foods
for a Better Body

On any given day, you face dozens of food and beverage choices. Eggs or a muffin? Coffee or tea? Club sandwich or soup and salad? Chicken or fish? Pizza or tacos? Beer or wine?

Each decision, big or small, can be part of your strategy to lose weight—and that doesn't mean living on carrot sticks and diet soda. On the contrary, any food is fair game, say experts. Foods you've been shunning aren't forbidden at all. And some foods you thought were low-cal may be delivering hidden fat and calories.

"You need to enjoy a variety of foods, and not too much or too little of any one food. Certainly go easy on high-calorie, high-fat foods. What counts is the fat and calories in your overall diet," says Roberta Duyff, R.D., a registered dietitian and food and nutrition consultant in St. Louis and author of *The American Dietetic Association's Complete Food and Nutrition Guide*, among other books.

Other dietitians agree.

"All kinds of negative feelings and behaviors come into play when you eat so-called bad foods," says Kim Galeaz,

R.D., a registered dietitian and food and nutrition consultant in Indianapolis. "Many people start to feel guilt, anxiety, and remorse. I'd like everyone to get over this 'good/bad' notion and start eating for enjoyment."

"It's easier to stick to a healthful eating plan when you include some favorites," says Elizabeth Ward, R.D., a registered dietitian in Stoneham, Massachusetts, and spokesperson for the American Dietetic Association. "Lose your all-or-nothing dieting mentality and gain some peace. Just because you ate more than you should at one meal doesn't spell dietary disaster. And keep in mind that you can eat more food when you include daily physical activity."

Use the following lists as they were intended—to guide you toward the better choices most of the time. "Best" selections are exceptionally helpful when you're trying to eat just a little leaner to counteract something with more calories you ate the previous day.

You can also use these examples to make trade-offs during the course of the day—a light dinner to compensate for selecting a special treat at lunch or celebrating with food at midday, for example.

Bagels, Breads, Rolls, and Muffins

Remember when dieters axed the bun and ate the burger? Back then, carbohydrates were the bad guys, and protein was all the rage. While convincing people that a high-protein diet was the answer to dieting woes, media hype unfairly bad-mouthed carbohydrates, especially those in bread and related foods. It still comes as a surprise to many people that bread can be one of the essentials in a lifelong weight-control routine.

The carbs in whole-grain breads are rich in nutrients. And these breads are high in hunger-satisfying fiber. On the other hand, white bread, white flour, pretzels, and white bagels run shy in nutrients, even though they're not loaded with fat.

For the bread you eat to qualify as the staff of life, you have to make the right choices when shopping. Here's what to look for.

Bread. Rich, variegated shades of tan, brown, and dark brown are often a clue that you're getting the whole-grain instead of the watered-down version. But they're not a foolproof indication. Molasses, caramel, and other coloring agents can help white bread masquerade as its healthier cousin. Make sure that the label confirms your choice. Look for words like "100 percent whole wheat." ("Wheat bread" doesn't guarantee whole grain.) And check that some type of whole grain flour is listed as the first ingredient.

Remember to have your bread sliced at the store. The employee can do it thinner than you can at home, which helps you control portion sizes. When you do cut your own bread, aim for 1-ounce slices. (If you know that it's a 20-ounce loaf, for instance, try to get 20 slices.) One ounce of bread counts as one serving of whole grains.

Bagels. Again, buy a variety. Even more important, pay attention to bagel size. Many bakery versions are the equivalent of five slices of bread and, at 5 five ounces, weigh in at around 390 calories. Depending on how you want to apportion your grain servings, cut these large bagels into halves or thirds. Bagels you buy frozen tend to be 2 ounces, the equivalent of two slices of bread. Watch out for some "bagel chips"—they are often heavily coated with oil or butter and not at all lean.

Muffins. They have such a healthy, homey image, yet too often they're high in fat. Some bakery muffins tip the scales at 15 grams of fat and 370 calories. Many fat-free ones are no calorie bargain either—larger muffins can weigh in with 350 to 600 calories, but very few nutrients.

Regard specialty muffins like chocolate chip with a wary eye. They're little more than chocolate cupcakes in disguise.

If you like to bake, try some of the lower-fat muffin mixes. By baking your own, you can control portion sizes. (You can even make mini-muffins.) When a box mix calls for oil, use half oil and half applesauce. To increase the nutritional value of the muffins, stir in grated carrots and some raisins. Both baking tricks increase flavor and moistness.

Dinner rolls and biscuits. The fancier they get, the fattier they are. Some of the worst offenders are the ready-to-

The Best Bagels, Breads, Rolls, and Muffins

To qualify as a healthful selection, bread items should have less than 4 grams of fat per ounce. Also, look for breads with at least 2 grams of fiber per serving.

Bread Item	Portion	Calories	Grams of Fat
Whole grain bread	1 slice (1 oz)	70	1.1
Whole wheat pita	1 small pita (1 oz)	74	0.7
Scandinavian flat bread	1 flat bread (1 oz)	104	0.4
Tomato and basil tortilla	1 tortilla (1½ oz)	110	1.0
Low-fat blueberry muffin	1 muffin (2 oz)	162	6.2
Pumpernickel bagel	1 bagel (4 oz)	250	1.0

bake rolls and biscuits in the dairy case and the frozen bake-and-serve products. Check the labels for fat and calories. As for frozen garlic bread, take care. You're staring at 360 calories and 17 grams of fat (for a 3½-ounce slice). Croissants can be even worse.

English muffins, French bread, and pita bread. These items tend to be very low in fat, with a reasonable number of calories. Try to find whole wheat versions. (But avoid the temptation to fill those "nooks and crannies" in the English muffins with puddles of butter!)

Apple butter and purees. These have not a lick of fat, but they do contain some vitamins and fiber. Buy them or make your own. To create an incredible puree even the kids will enjoy, scoop baked acorn squash from its shell and place in a food processor with a splash of milk and a sprinkle of ground cinnamon and brown sugar. Blend until smooth. Store in the refrigerator for up to a week. Use the same basic concept for cooked apples, pears, pumpkin, peaches, and more.

Weight-Friendly Substitutions

Traditional Scandinavian flat breads are easier to find than ever. Resembling thin crackers, these delightfully crisp breads are made with a combination of wheat, barley, potato, and rye flours. Serve them as the Scandinavians do—with soups, salads, and low-fat cheeses. They're fat-free, fiber rich, and naturally low in calories—just 104 per 1-ounce cracker.

If you can't imagine spaghetti, lasagna, or other Italian foods without garlic bread, try checking a bakery for ciabatta. This low-fat "Swiss cheese of breads" has large holes peppered throughout its cloud-soft interior and is so flavorful it doesn't need butter, margarine, or olive oil. Warm the loaf briefly in a hot oven to make the outside even crisper.

Some new products worth avoiding: pizza breads (such as cheese and pepperoni) and focaccia. Although focaccia is extremely popular, it's also high in fat.

Beverages

A lot of women don't keep track of beverages they drink, which can squelch their weight-control efforts like a tidal wave—especially since a can of soda contains 150 calories and nearly as much sugar as two candy bars.

Water is the one beverage that helps your weight-loss efforts. People who drink water before meals eat fewer calories and have an easier time taking off excess pounds. That's because water fills your stomach, so you don't eat as much.

When used appropriately, wet calories can help, not hinder, your body-shaping efforts. Here's how.

Shopping Smarts

For tips on buying milk and soy milk, see "Milk and Dairy," on page 77. Otherwise, follow these purchasing tips.

Water. Buy enough for a week. (If you drink tap water, fill four or five 20-ounce reusable sipper bottles and chill them in the refrigerator. Then carry water with you during the day.)

Still water is fine. If a little fizz helps you chug down more wet stuff, buy calorie-free flavored seltzer or club soda. Just avoid the ones that are heavy in sugar and calories. They hide nearly as many calories as regular soda.

Coffee and coffee drinks. True, coffee contributes only 5 calories—if you drink it black. The real damage, however, comes from specialty coffees—the lattes, mochas, cappuccinos, and other tall treats sold in coffee bars and shops. Choose poorly and you've just blown

The Best Beverages

Plain water is the best thing you can drink. Beverages that contain fat and sugar are the worst. Drinks that offer some nutrition in return for their caloric cost, such as an 8-ounce glass of skim milk, are also a wise choice. Serving sizes given here are typical for each drink.

Beverage	Serving Size	Calories	Grams of Fat
Still or sparkling water	8 oz	0	0.0
Unsweetened, flavored water	8 oz	0	0.0
Unsweetened, flavored iced tea	8 oz	5	0.0
Vegetable juice	8 oz	46	0.2
Calcium-fortified orange juice	8 oz	120	0.7
Grape juice	8 oz	127	0.2

your dessert calories for the next month. An 8-ounce regular café mocha splashes in at 493 calories and 49 grams of fat. Order it with nonfat milk and sans whipped cream (substitute the foam from steaming the nonfat milk), add artificial sweetener, and sneak by with just 120 calories.

Iced tea. If you're going to drink iced tea, drink plain, old-fashioned iced tea—made from tea bags and flavored with lemon. It has just 2 calories, plus you get plenty of water in the bargain. A 16-ounce bottle of flavored, sweetened iced tea is the equivalent of a soda.

Juices. With few exceptions, juice is mainly sugar. Two exceptions: Calcium-fortified orange juice helps satisfy the essential bone-building calcium requirement for women who don't drink milk. And vegetable juice offers a wide variety of nutrients for few calories (46 calories in 8 ounces).

Alcohol. Experts agree that people who drink red wine in moderation seem to enjoy some protection against heart disease. Still, if you're watching your weight, that benefit comes at a caloric price—7 calories per gram of alcohol, or about 103 calories per 5-ounce glass. If you drink wine out of goblets, used in many homes and restaurants, you'll consume even more. And if you drink hard liquor, like gin or vodka, you'll quaff 97 calories or more in a shot, depending on the proof, plus whatever mixer you choose. Liqueur (like coffee liqueur) is even higher, at 160 calories per 1½-ounce shot. As for those fruity tropical drinks like piña coladas—you might as well be drinking a chocolate milkshake.

If you don't like alcohol, both black and green teas, which have zero calories, may provide heart-protecting benefits similar to red wine. And if you do drink, keep the calories from alcohol to a minimum.

Weight-Friendly Substitutions

If you just have to have a higher-calorie beverage, try the following substitutions.

- Instead of regular lemonade (99 calories per 8 ounces), substitute artificially sweetened lemonade drink (5 calories).
- Instead of wine (103 calories per 5 ounces), have a wine spritzer (62 calories per 5 ounces).
- Instead of a chocolate milkshake (430 calories for 12 ounces), order a café mocha skim, no whipped cream (120 calories per 12 ounces).

Burgers and Hot Dogs

If these foods appeared only on special occasions, they wouldn't pose too much of a weight problem. Unfortunately, in many homes they've turned into everyday guests.

The Best Burgers and Hot Dogs

Your best bets are burgers made from ground top round or sirloin or ground chicken or turkey, with no more than 10 grams of fat and 260 calories per 3-ounce cooked patty. Hot dogs aren't nutrient dense—eat them only occasionally and aim for the lower-fat versions (beef, pork, poultry, or veggie), with no more than 7 grams of fat.

Burger or Hot Dog	Portion	Calories	Grams of Fat
Fat-free hot dog	1 hot dog	40	0.0
Turkey hot dog	1 hot dog	85	6.0
Light hot dog	1 hot dog	110	8.4
Veggie dog	1 hot dog	118	7.0
Lean smoked sausage (broiled)	3 oz	120	3.6
Soy/veggie burger	1 patty (about 3 oz)	137	4.1
Burger made from ground top round (broiled, no bun)	3 oz	153	4.2
Burger made from ground sirloin (broiled, no bun)	3 oz	166	6.1
Small hamburger (fast-food)	1 burger	260	9.0

Hot dogs offer protein and little else (except fat to the tune of 16 grams for a regular frank). Burgers can be better nutrition-wise, pairing iron, vitamin B_{12}, and zinc with their protein. But they're no dietary bargain either, given choices like the McDonald's Quarter Pounder with 21 grams of fat.

Luckily, you don't have to give up hot dogs and hamburgers altogether. You just need to be more discerning when choosing them. Here are things to keep in mind at the store.

Burgers. Take a good look at that package of "lean" ground beef. What you really want to know is *how* lean. Regular ground beef is about 73 percent lean (which means 27 percent fat)—a 3-ounce cooked patty has 18 grams of fat. Ground round (85 percent lean) is a little better. But ground sirloin (90 percent) and ground top round (97 percent) are wiser choices. A cooked ground sirloin patty has 6 grams of fat—one-third of what that regular ground beef gives you.

If you can't find really lean ground meat, ask the butcher to grind some sirloin or top round for you. (Make sure he trims off excess fat first.) An alternative is to use ground turkey breast or chicken breast—or to mix either with some ground beef to lower the fat content. Be aware that meat marked simply "ground turkey" or "ground chicken" contains dark meat and skin in addition to breast meat, so it's not nearly as low in fat as plain ground breast.

Grill or broil your burgers so any fat in them can drip off. (Or use a ridged grill pan made for the stove top.) If you must use a regular skillet, blot the cooked burgers with paper towels to remove surface fat.

Hot dogs. Your best choices in hot dogs are those with 3 grams or less of fat. Look for the words "reduced fat," "low fat," or "fat-free" on the label. Don't think that because it says turkey or chicken on the package, it's automatically low in fat. Regular turkey and chicken dogs can still pack 6 to 9 grams of fat each.

Weight-Friendly Substitutions

Try meatless vegetable patties. Although not necessarily fat-free—they range from zero to 8 grams of fat—they're very low in saturated fat and have no cholesterol. Look for plain burger flavor, spicy black bean, mushroom, sautéed onion, garden vegetable, and more. Some are even made with soy protein, which has been said to lower one's risk of developing cancer, osteoporosis, and heart disease.

Besides ready-made patties, various all-vegetable meat substitutes come in 1-pound logs so you can shape your own burgers or hot dog look-alikes.

Look for veggie hot dogs, many of which have 7 grams of fat or less. Their main benefit is soy protein. Also try low-fat sausages, which have lots of seasonings to compensate for the fat that has been removed. Serve any type of burger or hot dog with mayo-Dijon spread.

Cereals

Cold or hot, cereal is a great way to start your day. Studies show that women who skip or skimp on breakfast tend to nibble more during the mid and late morning, perhaps eating even more calories than if they'd eaten breakfast in the first place.

Of course, a breakfast of bacon and eggs won't help your weight-loss goals. Served with buttered toast, fried eggs and two strips of bacon will gird you with 28 grams of fat and 395 calories. In contrast, a bowl of bran flakes, a ½ cup of fat-free milk, and a ½ cup of sliced strawberries will supply 1 gram of fat and 200 calories.

Except for some granolas, which may contain saturated vegetable fat like coconut oil, most ready-to-eat cereals are low in calories from fat. For the most part, cereal serves as one of your best sources of complex carbohydrates (which, say nutrition experts, should account for 55 to 60 percent of your daily calories).

Some cereals provide as much as 8 to 12 grams of

The Best Cereals

Most cereals are low in fat and can also be a source of many vitamins, minerals, and fiber. A good cereal supplies at least 5 grams of fiber per serving. Focus on whole grain cereals and those with bran or fortified with fiber. If you like granola, choose low-fat versions, and compare the number of calories per serving. Read labels, and select cereals that contain the lowest amounts of sugar per serving.

Cereal	Portion	Calories	Grams of Fat	Grams of Fiber
Bran cereal with extra fiber	½ cup	50	0.5	13.3
100 percent bran	⅓ cup	80	0.5	8.0
Instant oatmeal with bran and raisins	1 packet (1.4 oz), prepared	158	1.9	5.5
Unsweetened shredded wheat	2 biscuits	160	0.5	5.0
Raisin bran	1 cup	190	1.0	8.0
Spoon-size wheat cereal	½ cup	133	0.0	2.7
Wheat bran flakes with dried fruit and nuts	1 cup	210	3.0	5.0

fiber—about a third of the 25 to 35 grams a day experts recommend. Bran cereals have the highest amounts. Overall, a diet high in fiber can help control your weight and lower your cholesterol. To reap all the benefits of fiber, vary your choices of whole-grain cereal from day to day.

Fortified breakfast cereals may supply a significant percent of your Daily Value of some vitamins and minerals, including B vitamins (like folic acid) and iron. Some are calcium-fortified, helping you maintain strong bones. Topping your cereal with milk or yogurt increases that benefit.

Here's how to make cereal part of your weight-smart breakfast.

Shopping Smarts

Finding packaged cereals with the least fat and fewest calories—and the most fiber—is easy: Read the ingredient list and Nutrition Facts information on the box. Pay attention to serving sizes: They vary from ½ to 1 cup or more.

Ready-to-eat cereal. Ready-to-eat cold cereal is a calorie bargain—provided you watch out for added sugars in presweetened cereals. To keep the number of calories down, don't get into the habit of adding a spoonful or two of sugar on your own.

Cooked cereal. Start with the best known—oatmeal, cream of wheat, and grits. Then look for other varieties, such as buckwheat, barley, oat bran, or a mixture of whole grains. Quick-cooking and instant varieties save time— just add water or milk, heat, and eat. (If you use milk, make it with low-fat or fat-free for fewer calories.)

Cheese and Cheese Dishes

A compact form of milk, cheese has a similar nutritional makeup—plenty of protein and calcium and a good supply of riboflavin. But a serving of cheese also has more fat and cholesterol than a 1-cup serving of milk does. Cheese makers offer fat-free or reduced-fat versions of many pop-

The Best Cheeses

USDA experts consider a serving of cheese to be 1½ ounces of natural cheese (like Cheddar) or 2 ounces of processed cheese (like American). But Nutrition Facts labels list a serving of cheese as 1 ounce. So to keep things simple, that's the benchmark used here. By law, low-fat varieties have 3 grams of fat or less per serving, fat-free have less than 0.5 gram of fat per serving, and reduced-fat cheese has at least 25 percent less fat per serving than traditional cheese.

Cheese	Portion	Calories	Grams of Fat
Fat-free Parmesan cheese	2 tsp	20	0.0
Parmesan cheese	2 tsp	20	1.5
Fat-free cream cheese	1 oz	30	0.0
Fat-free mozzarella	1 oz	35	0.0
Low-fat American processed cheese	1 slice	40	1.0
Fat-free Cheddar cheese	1 oz	45	0.0
Low-fat Cheddar cheese	1 oz	50	1.5
Low-fat mozzarella	1 oz	50	1.5
Reduced-fat feta	1 oz	50	3.0
Reduced-fat cheese spread	1 oz	60	3.0
Low-fat ricotta	¼ cup	70	3.0
Fat-free cottage cheese	½ cup	90	0.0
Low-fat (1 to 2 percent) cottage cheese	½ cup	90	1.5

ular types of cheese, including cream cheese and Brie. If you prefer the flavor and cooking qualities of full-fat cheeses, eat small portions so that you can keep your fat and calorie intake within "budget." Grate or shred cheese, rather than use slices or chunks, to make a smaller amount go further.

Shopping Smarts

Low-fat cheeses are good sources of calcium. Whether you buy regular or reduced-fat cheese, in chunks or shredded, check the Nutrition Facts label, especially if you're salt-sensitive. The sodium content will vary. Also, cheese is perishable, so check expiration dates.

If you buy sliced cheese or wedges at the deli counter, feel free to request nutrition information. By law, it must be available.

Here's how to select the low-fat cheeses that best meet your needs.

Cheddar, Swiss, and other aged cheeses. You'll find fat-free or reduced-fat versions of some, but not all, types of aged cheese. The melting qualities, texture, and flavor differ from brand to brand. Some brands work better than others as substitutes for full-fat cheese. In general, low-fat cheeses have better cooking qualities than their fat-free counterparts.

For pizza, lasagna, and other Italian dishes, look for low-fat or fat-free mozzarella. For a fun snack, try fat-free string cheese, which is a variation of mozzarella.

Processed cheese. American cheese, cheese spreads, and other pasteurized blends aren't ripened or aged. As a result, they don't have the same distinct flavor and texture as aged cheese. But they're versatile and keep longer than aged cheese.

Cottage cheese, ricotta, and cream cheese. Often viewed as a diet food, cottage cheese may not be quite as low calorie as many people think—it depends on the fat content. For the lowest fat and calorie counts, look for fat-free or 1 percent milk-fat cottage cheese. For salad dressings and dips, whip fat-free cottage cheese as a thickener or as a substitute for sour cream. Reduced-fat or fat-free ricotta works well in baked dishes, such as lasagna and pastitsio (a Greek version of lasagna).

Cream cheese is very high in fat; look for reduced-fat and fat-free types. Some varieties are herb-, fruit-, or salmon-flavored. These are nice for dips as well as spreads. Don't count on cream cheese for calcium, though—it supplies little.

Soy cheese. Made from soy protein, soy cheese (sometimes called tofu cheese) is a lower-fat, cholesterol-free alternative to dairy cheese. It doesn't taste much like cheese, however. Experiment to see if it appeals to you.

Weight-Friendly Substitutions

These low-fat kitchen tips can help you enjoy the flavor and texture of cheese without overdosing on fat and calories.

- In cheese spreads, extend a small amount of stronger-flavored cheese—such as Asiago, blue cheese, feta, sharp Cheddar, or Romano cheese—with fat-free yogurt or cottage cheese.
- Reduced-fat and fat-free cheeses melt better if you layer them between other foods or cover the dish while it's baking.
- Use sliced soy cheese in sandwiches and lasagna and other baked dishes. Or shred it for casseroles and salad or soup toppers.
- Substitute soft tofu (a block of milky white soybean curd) for cream cheese in dips, medium-soft tofu in cheesecake, and sliced firm tofu in sandwiches.
- Try Neufchâtel cheese, light cream cheese, and fat-free cream cheese in cheesecake.

Chicken and Turkey

Poultry is loaded with protein, an essential nutrient that repairs tissue, bolsters immunity, and helps keep your heart beating and your brain cells firing. While many other protein foods, such as beef and pork, can be high in fat, chicken and turkey shine because they're easily slimmed down by removing the skin, either before or after cooking. Three ounces of grilled or roasted skinless chicken breast (a serving about the size of a deck of cards) gives you 53 percent of the Daily Value for protein and just 3 grams of fat. It also supplies generous amounts of niacin, vitamin B_6, and iron.

Shopping Smarts

Years ago, buying and cooking poultry was simple: You bought a whole bird, then either roasted it or cut it up for other dishes. Today you can buy chicken part by part, with or without skin, with or without bones, raw or precooked. Here's a look at how to make the best of what's available.

Boneless, skinless chicken breasts and thighs. Cut boneless breast meat into strips, then keep a package or two in your freezer. It will come in handy for stir-fries, fajitas, and chow mein. Both breasts and thighs are good in most sauté recipes because they add little (if any) fat to whatever sauce you have in the pan.

Chicken breasts, legs, or thighs on the bone, with skin. These pieces are great for marinating and grilling because they hold in flavor and moisture. If you're going to baste the meat with a sauce such as barbecue sauce, remove the skin first to allow the sauce to cook in and flavor the meat more fully. Otherwise, remove it before eating.

Skinless chicken breasts or thighs on the bone. This type of chicken is best for oven frying or for skillet dishes.

Whole chicken. Roasting chickens are meant for roasting, not frying or grilling. The whole bird generally has more fat than individual pieces without skin, so roast it on a rack to allow the fat to run off, and remove the skin before serving.

Chicken lunchmeat. All chicken lunchmeat isn't created equal, with some brands packing in as much fatty filler as bologna. Select lunchmeat with 2 grams of fat or less per ounce. And if you're cutting back on sodium for any reason, bear in mind that most lunchmeats are high in sodium.

Turkey breast. Choose the real thing, not the processed version. (Processed turkey is a combination of pressed white and dark meat, and it's loaded with salt.) Roast a turkey covered to lock in the moisture, and enjoy the leftovers on salads and in sandwiches.

Turkey cutlets. These are perfect for grilling, sautéing, and baking. Cutlets cook quickly and need some moisture, so marinate them, then baste with your favorite nonfat sauce—such as barbecue, teriyaki, or sweet-and-sour— throughout cooking.

Ground turkey. Regular ground turkey is no leaner than most ground beef, so reach for the extra-lean version. Three ounces of regular ground turkey has more than 11 grams of fat, while the same amount of extra-lean light meat ground turkey has just 2.6 grams.

Turkey sausage, lunchmeat, and hot dogs. Choose carefully. Consumers assume that these items are low in fat, but many are not. Read the label to be certain that you're getting a lower-fat version with less than 2 grams of fat per ounce.

New Foods to Try

Try Rock Cornish game hens, pheasant, and quail. Game hens are available at many supermarkets, and you can ask a butcher to order pheasant or quail. Although they cost more, these low-fat, high-nutrition birds are a unique taste sensation. Three skinless ounces of each (about the size of

The Best Chicken and Turkey Selections

Unadorned, chicken and turkey are low in fat and calories. But how we order or prepare the two—fried, barbecued, roasted, or souped up in dozens of ways—can drastically alter them (for better or worse). Here's a look at how some popular entrées measure up in calorie and fat content. (A healthy poultry entrée should contain no more than 500 calories and 15 grams of fat.) The portions listed are typical servings for each dish.

Entrée	Portion	Calories	Grams of Fat
Sliced, skinless roasted turkey	3 oz	133	2.7
Barbecued, skinless chicken breast	3 oz, with 2 Tbsp barbecue sauce	167	3.7
Grilled chicken kabobs	2 skewers	170	4.0
Lemon turkey cutlet	1 cutlet, sautéed with lemon and herbs	186	5.3
Oven-fried, skinless chicken	1 leg and thigh, with buttermilk and bread crumb coating	229	8.8
Grilled, skinless chicken breast	½ breast (3 oz), with rosemary and black olives	245	8.0
Chicken fajitas	2 fajitas with grilled chicken and peppers	318	5.0

your palm) has a skimpy 3.3 grams of fat. And there's no need to seek out exotic recipes for these birds: They can be roasted just as you would a chicken or a turkey. For a low-fat, high-flavor treat, try pheasant cacciatore, prepared with mushrooms, onions, and tomatoes and seasoned with Italian herbs such as garlic, basil, and oregano.

Two other members of the poultry family—duck and goose—are high in fat. Save them for special occasions.

Condiments and Spreads

A stroll through any supermarket shows that we're a nation of condiment lovers. Besides ketchup, mustard, and mayonnaise, there are marinades, sauces, spreads, relishes, dips, salsas, mustards, and more.

By definition, a condiment is "a savory, piquant, spicy, or salty accompaniment to food." Condiments and spreads concentrate flavor—and sometimes considerable fat and calories, if you're not careful.

If you're like a lot of people, you probably rely on condiments for breakfast, lunch, dinner, and parties. By day's end, you can accumulate a fair amount of fat and calories from condiments and spreads alone. Chosen wisely, however, condiments can add excitement and flavor for very little fat and few calories. Here's how.

Shopping Smarts

If you've been trying to lose weight, you probably switched to fat-free or reduced-fat mayonnaise and "diet" margarine years ago. And you probably already read food labels closely for fat and calorie counts. Here are a few category-specific tips to help make the most of the zillion choices in the condiments and spreads aisle.

Fat-free or reduced-fat mayonnaises. Per tablespoon, low-fat (or light) brands contain 50 fewer calories and 6 grams of fat less than regular mayonnaise, and fat-free varieties run about 90 fewer calories and 11 grams of fat less. For a flavor boost, stir in some minced garlic or onion from the spice rack.

Butters, margarines, and margarine-like spreads. Just 1 tablespoon of butter or full-fat margarine contains about 12 grams of fat and 108 calories. As a table spread, "calorie-reduced" or "light" tub margarine-like spread is your best bet, saving you 8.5 grams of fat and 73 calories per tablespoon. Try different brands to find the flavor and texture that appeal most to you. Don't use reduced-fat spreads and margarines for cooking, though—they're high in water, so they won't brown foods, and they can ruin baked goods.

Look for margarine or margarine-like spreads made with olive or canola oil. These products are higher in monounsaturated fats and are less likely to clog coronary arteries than other vegetable oils. Also, look for varieties that are free of trans fatty acids (by-products of the manufacturing process that make margarine solid at room temperature and affect your heart like saturated fats do).

Mustards. Brown, yellow, smooth, coarse—most contain a scant 4 to 10 calories per teaspoon and virtually no fat. Be adventurous—try Dijon, Parisian, and stone-ground varieties, as well as those with added herbs. For a sweet touch, try honey mustard, but be aware that 1 tablespoon has 30 calories, not 4 or 5. So spread thinly.

Tartar sauce, horseradish, and relish. Once you've switched to fish without butter, lean roast beef, and fat-free hot dogs, you don't want to cancel out your calorie-saving efforts by smothering them in high-fat condiments. You won't go wrong here—provided you look for low-fat tartar sauce and prepared horseradish, not the cream sauce variety. No luck? Just mix some pickle relish or prepared horseradish with a tablespoon or two of fat-free mayo.

Jam, jelly, and marmalade. Fruit spreads are pure sugar—but not off-limits. Substituting 1 teaspoon of jam or marmalade for 1 teaspoon of butter or margarine on breads, bagels, and English muffins cuts calories from your spread by more than half—from 36 to 16. The key is to buy the best strawberry preserves, orange marmalade, raspberry jam—whatever is your favorite—and then enjoy just a little. Or, for a lower-calorie, less sugary alternative, try fruit butter.

Bottled sauces. From good old Texas-style barbecue sauce to Oriental duck sauce, you'll find a virtual United Nations of flavor enhancers available for meat, chicken, and fish: steak sauce, teriyaki, miso (a soy product), hoisin, Szechuan—plus the standard soy sauce and ketchup. Calorically speaking, they're all pretty low—4 to 8 calories per teaspoon—and they ring up a scant portion of 1 gram of fat (compare that with Mornay sauce, at triple the calories and at least 2 grams of fat per teaspoon). Slathered on lean beef, pork, or poultry, these sauces will serve your weight-loss effort well.

Salsas. They're cooked or fresh mixtures of tomatoes, sweet peppers, hot peppers, and onions. Traditionally, there were just two salsa staples: "salsa cruda," uncooked tomato-based salsa, and "salsa verde," green salsa made from raw tomatillos, green chili peppers, and cilantro. Today the selection is wider, with varieties that are chunky or spicy or that use all kinds of vegetables or even fruit.

Spoon salsa on baked potatoes instead of sour cream, spread it on steamed broccoli and cauliflower, drop it by the spoonful onto grilled chicken, fish, and veggie burgers.

Most salsas are fat-free, but double-check the label and bypass any laced with cheese or oil.

New Foods to Try

Consider these condiment concepts in your shape-up efforts.

The Best Condiments and Spreads

As a rule, try to limit the calories from condiments at any one meal to 50 or fewer. Be especially careful with jams and jellies (40 to 50 calories per tablespoon) and peanut butter (90 calories per tablespoon). If you use no more than a couple of teaspoons of these spreads, you can enjoy toast, bagels, and crackers without going overboard on fat and calories.

Condiment	Portion	Calories	Grams of Fat
Tabasco (hot pepper) sauce	1 tsp	1	0.0
Fresh lemon juice	1 Tbsp	4	0.0
Thick and chunky salsa	1 Tbsp	5	0.0
Prepared horseradish	1 Tbsp	6	0.0
Fat-free mayonnaise	1 Tbsp	10	0.0
Sugar-free jam	1 Tbsp	10	0.0
Yellow mustard	1 Tbsp	12	0.0
Apple butter	1 Tbsp	15	0.0
Bean spread	1 Tbsp	15	0.0
Cocktail sauce	1 Tbsp	15	0.0
Ketchup	1 Tbsp	16	0.0
Sweet pickle relish	1 Tbsp	20	0.0
"Light" tub margarine-like spread	1 Tbsp	35	3.5

Margarine-like sprays. For most of these sprays, the main ingredient is soybean oil. These brilliant inventions tally no calories or fat for the spritz necessary to coat toast, an English muffin, air-popped popcorn, or steamed veggies.

Creamy mustard blends. A mustard-mayo blend gives mayonnaise lovers lots of the creamy taste, with just 5 calories and zero grams of fat per teaspoon (enough for a sandwich).

Soy butters. Made from roasted soybeans, reduced-fat soy butter has about one-third the fat of peanut butter. When it's paired with their favorite jam, jelly, or fruit butter, even your kids will eat it.

Ethnic sauces. To lend an ethnic flair to your family's standard meat-and-rice dishes, try a Thai or Jamaican sauce. These are usually found on the grocery shelf next to the soy sauce.

Fruit salsas. These salsas make delightful accompaniments for chicken, fish, and all sorts of vegetables. Start with mango salsa and grilled chicken—there will be no going back.

Bean spreads and hummus. Shop around for bean-salsa dips or hummus (a savory combination of chickpeas and sesame butter). When spread on fat-free chips, low-fat crackers, or toasted pita bread, these savory spreads are a valuable alternative to cheese spreads. For the best bet, read labels.

Desserts

Experts say that for long-term weight control, you don't need to swear off dessert. You'll only feel deprived and go whole-hog when you do give in.

Chosen wisely, dessert can contribute nutrients that you need. Pudding made from a mix with low-fat or fat-free milk contributes calcium, for example.

The keys: Make dessert calories count. Keep an eye on fat and sugar. And rein in the portions.

Be aware that "low-fat" and "fat-free" aren't a license for second helpings. Eating twice as much can easily negate the benefit of choosing a low-fat version. Also, many reduced-fat treats—with their added sugar—more than make up for the calories from fat. The fat-free versions may have more calories than the regular versions.

Shopping Smarts

If time is short, buy convenience products. For products that promise to be low-fat or fat-free, check the Nutrition Facts on the back of the package and compare the calorie and fat content with that of regular products. They may not necessarily have fewer calories.

To prepare low-calorie, low-fat desserts from scratch, stock the staples below.

Pantry staples. If you like to bake, keep these items on hand.

- Whole wheat flour, oatmeal, and other whole grains, such as barley flour (to boost the fiber content in baked goods)
- Low-fat or fat-free dairy products for baked dishes (You can substitute fat-free evaporated milk and buttermilk for cream.)
- Naturally sweetened fruit spreads, applesauce, and prune butter (to replace part of the fat in baked goods).
- Sugar substitutes (Read the tips for use on the package. Those with aspartame aren't appropriate for cooked or baked desserts.)
- Vegetable oil spray (to coat baking pans)

Mixes. For quick homemade desserts, look for mixes with less fat or sugar: low-fat and sugar-free pudding mix, low-fat cake mix, low-fat brownie mix, low-fat cheesecake mix, angel food cake mix, and sugar-free gelatin, to name just a few.

Frozen desserts. Try lower-fat and fat-free varieties of ice cream as well as frozen yogurt, ices, and sorbet.

Packaged treats. Tuck the following products into your shopping cart.

- Vanilla wafers, gingersnaps, or graham crackers. Enjoy as is or use for crumb crusts.
- Low-fat crumb crusts. Fill with low-fat pudding.
- Angel food cake from the bakery department. Just slice and spread fruit or frozen yogurt between the layers.
- Low-fat, sugar-free cookies. Read the label to see if they're really low calorie.

Weight-Friendly Substitutions

To make your desserts more weight-friendly, try cutting back on high-fat and sugary ingredients. Be aware, though: In many desserts, especially baked desserts, substitutions affect the texture, volume, and flavor of the end result. Experiment a bit to get results that satisfy you.

For baked desserts:

- Replace up to half the fat with an equal amount of fruit puree, such as mashed banana, applesauce, or prune butter. You can expect especially good results in bar and drop cookies.
- Experiment with vanilla yogurt in place of butter or margarine in muffins and quick breads. Use reduced-fat cream cheese in cheesecake.
- Instead of buttery cake, prepare angel food cake, which is made with egg whites and no fat.
- Use fresh fruit or fruit canned in juices, rather than syrup, in fruit crisps and cobblers.

For toppings:

- Instead of frosting, top cakes with fresh sliced fruit, lemon yogurt, or frozen yogurt.
- For a thick sauce, puree fruit with a little juice to the consistency you want. Try different types of fruits (mango, kiwifruit, blackberry, or apricots) or a mixture. If you wish, thin the sauce with a splash of white wine.

The Best Desserts

You can have any dessert you like—provided you don't eat the whole thing, don't eat it every day, and don't have it several times a day. That said, these choices have less fat and fewer calories. Select pre-pared desserts or recipes that have 25 percent fewer calories per serving than the traditional versions. If you can find desserts that are also low-fat, that's even better.

Dessert	Portion	Calories	Grams of Fat
Poached fruit topped with toasted oatmeal	1 peach and 2 Tbsp oatmeal	55	0.0
Fat-free pudding (prepared from a dry mix with fat-free milk)	½ cup	70	0.0
Meringue cookies	4 cookies (about ¾ oz total)	73	0.0
Sorbet	½ cup	80	0.0
Angel food cake with fresh fruit	1 slice (¹⁄₁₂ of cake)	85	0.0
Biscotti	1 cookie (about ¾ oz)	100	3.0
Low-fat frozen yogurt	½ cup	110	2.5
Gingersnaps	4 cookies (about 1 oz total)	120	2.5
Strawberries with low-fat frozen yogurt	¼ cup sliced berries with ½ cup frozen yogurt	122	2.5

- Dust cakes with confectioners' sugar mixed with instant coffee, spices, or cocoa.

For crusts:
- Prepare desserts with a single, not a double, crust. Or use a low-fat prepared crumb crust.
- For a homemade crumb crust, coat the pan with vegetable oil spray, then dust it with graham cracker crumbs.
- Top fruit crisp or pie with rolled oats, instead of a pastry crust.

For custard or pudding desserts:
- Prepare effortless puddings with a fat-free or low-fat mix. Layer them with fruit for creamy parfaits, or pour them into a low-calorie crust.
- Prepare custard or rice pudding with low-fat milk and egg whites or egg substitute. Flavor with cinnamon and cranberries. Serve topped with freshly sliced fruit.

For any desserts:
- Enhance the flavor with fresh ginger, grated citrus rind, mint, and spices. Cut back on sugar, honey, and other sweeteners.
- Substitute low-fat or nonfat plain yogurt—cup for cup—in recipes that call for sour cream.
- For cakes and other baked chocolate desserts, replace melted chocolate with cocoa powder. Shave a little chocolate on top for flavor but few calories.

Eggs and Egg Dishes

Sitting unadorned in your refrigerator door, a large egg contains about 5 grams of fat and 75 calories, including just 1½ grams of saturated fat. The problem is not fat or calories but cholesterol. Experts advise limiting intake of dietary cholesterol to 300 milligrams a day.

Eggs have more cholesterol than just about any food— 213 milligrams in one large egg, all of it in the yolk. Experts recommend limiting your intake to four whole eggs or egg yolks a week from all kinds of food—omelets, quiche, and so forth. Be aware that eggs are also used in baked goods and mayonnaise. (On the other hand, you can eat all the egg whites you want—they have zero cholesterol.)

As you're rationing your egg yolks, you also want to keep a lid on high-fat, high-calorie ingredients added during the preparation of egg dishes. Butter or margarine, mayonnaise, cream, and cheese can add significant amounts of fat and calories. With careful planning, you can prepare eggs-traordinary meals while watching fat and calories.

Shopping Smarts

Basically, you have two choices when buying eggs—whole eggs and egg substitutes. Here's what to use and when.

Whole eggs. Four jumbo eggs equal five large eggs or six small eggs. Obviously, jumbo eggs have more of everything—calories and nutrients—than smaller varieties. Most recipes are written using large eggs.

Egg substitutes. These are blends of egg whites, nonfat milk, cornstarch, and vegetable oil, plus some vitamins and minerals. They look like raw scrambled eggs, and they have no cholesterol and as few as 35 calories per ¼ cup. Check the Nutrition Facts panel for calorie and nutrient content since some have fat, but others don't.

You'll find egg substitutes in the frozen foods and re-frigerated cases in your supermarket. You can use them to replace some or all of the whole eggs or egg yolks in your breakfast or in baked goods. Once the package is opened, keep it refrigerated and use the substitute within 3 days.

Egg replacers. For totally vegetarian meals, health food stores often sell egg replacers, a mixture of potato starch, flour, and leavening, which can substitute for whole eggs or egg whites. Just be aware that without egg whites for consistency, dishes made with egg-free products may lack the texture and flavor you expect from eggs.

Weight-Friendly Substitutions

The easiest way to work eggs into your menu without going overboard on calories or cholesterol is to prepare them without added fat.

The Best Egg Selections

Eggs are a good source of protein and average about 75 calories and 5 grams of fat apiece—without added or accompanying fat. If you're watching your cholesterol intake, consider that a whole egg supplies 213 milligrams of cholesterol. Experts advise consuming no more than four eggs or egg yolks per week. Keep in mind that many egg dishes can be made with low-fat or cholesterol-free ingredients.

Egg	Portion	Calories	Grams of Fat
Scrambled egg substitute	equivalent to 1 egg	35	0.0
Poached egg (yolk well-cooked)	1 egg	75	5.0
Hard-cooked egg	1 egg	78	5.3
Egg salad made with fat-free mayonnaise	½ cup	98	5.3
Vegetable omelet made with egg substitute	substitute equivalent to 2 eggs	125	4.0

For breakfast eggs:

- Extend scrambled eggs by adding chopped, steamed vegetables just before the eggs are done cooking, and use one egg per person.
- To lighten up scrambled eggs, blend in a stiffly beaten egg white or pureed nonfat cottage cheese.
- Cook scrambled eggs and omelettes in a nonstick pan that has been lightly coated with vegetable oil spray.
- Prepare a hard-cooked egg instead of a fried egg for breakfast. To save time in the morning, prepare eggs the night before, then refrigerate.

For egg salad:

- Blend the eggs with thick low-fat yogurt, pureed cottage cheese, or fat-free mayonnaise. Add a touch of dry mustard, horseradish, paprika, or chives. Prepare the yolks of deviled eggs the same way.
- To extend egg salad, mix in chopped celery or red or green bell pepper and serve it nestled in a sliced whole tomato.
- Substitute chopped firm tofu for hard-cooked eggs for a mock egg salad.

In other dishes:

- Replace whole eggs with egg whites or egg substitute. As a rule of thumb, two egg whites or ¼ cup of egg substitute replaces one whole egg. This tip is as good for omelettes as it is for baked goods.
- Use one whole egg and substitute two egg whites for the other egg when a recipe calls for two eggs or more.
- For totally egg-free baked goods, substitute half a small, ripe mashed banana or ¼ cup pureed fruit for each egg.

Fast Food

Believe it or not, you can still eat smart at fast-food restaurants (especially if they're not the mainstay of your diet.) Alongside the standard greasy, salty fare are healthier options. Your mission is to seek them out—and recognize them when you see them. Here's how.

Shopping Smarts

Ask for nutrition information for the food served. Many places either have brochures on hand or post the information on the wall. Most of the major chains also have that type of information posted on their Web sites. Print out those pages and keep them in your car. That way you can make your choice before you even walk in the door.

If you have to wing it, focus on bread, vegetables, fruit, and milk. Pass up pastries, sugar, and fries. For example, instead of fatty fries, order nutrient-dense vegetables, like a side salad. A carton of milk would meet your dairy needs. Juice is better than soda.

Burgers. "Mega," "super," and "jumbo" portions give you mega fat and calories. Instead, think in terms of reasonable portions—kid size, if necessary. The regular hamburgers at McDonald's and Burger King have half the calories and a third of the fat of their overstuffed big brothers. Finally, ask for burgers to be prepared without special sauces or to have the sauce served on the side.

Mexican. Establishments like Taco Bell offer items featuring refried beans, a fiber-filled change from meat. You're better off choosing a bean burrito, with 12 grams of fat, than a Big Beef Burrito Supreme, which weighs in at 23 grams of fat.

Chicken and fish. These items aren't always a healthier choice than burgers. Pay attention to how they're cooked. Are they grilled without extra sauces and toppings? Or are they breaded and fried? If chicken comes with the skin on, remove it and throw away lots of fat. (At Kentucky Fried Chicken, for instance, a roast chicken breast without skin has 4 grams of fat; one with skin has 11 grams.)

Baked potatoes. Get a plain spud and top it with healthy salad bar choices like peas, onions, tomatoes, and

The Best Fast Food

Think small, not supersize. Keep it plain—not cheesy, saucy, or smothered. Look for lower-fat choices.

Fast Food	Portion	Calories	Grams of Fat
Soft taco	1 taco	220	10.0
Bagel (with 2 Tbsp fat-free cream cheese)	1 bagel (2½ oz)	225	1.1
Grilled steak soft taco	1 taco	230	10.0
Baked potato (with ½ cup broccoli and 2 pats of butter)	1 potato	244	8.5
Small hamburger with bun (without condiments)	1 hamburger	260	9.0
Sub sandwich with lean turkey, ham, and vegetables (no mayo)	1 sandwich (6 in)	280	5.0
English muffin sandwich (with egg, Canadian bacon, American cheese, and buttered muffin)	1 sandwich	290	12.0
Grilled chicken sandwich (without mayonnaise)	1 sandwich	370	9.0
Bean burrito	1 burrito	380	12.0
Pancakes and syrup	1 serving (3 pancakes)	440	9.0

green peppers. Or order a small bowl of chili to top your spud. At 7 grams of fat, it's a better choice than asking for the menu-item chili and cheese baked potato (22 grams).

Salads and sandwiches. Subway has a wide variety of salads with fat-free dressings. (Try the roasted chicken breast salad: It has 162 calories and 4 grams of fat.) Many bagel places feature bagel sandwiches as well as soups.

Accompaniments. Ask about low-fat versions of mayonnaise, salad dressing, and milk. They may be available, just not listed on the menu. You'll find low-fat chips and lots of vegetable choices for sandwiches at Subway, for instance.

New Fast-Food Restaurants to Try

There's more out there than burger joints. Here are some places to look for good food in a flash.

Bagel shops. Many bagel shops offer lunch items. Lots of lower-fat options are available, like lean lunchmeat, smoked salmon, and hummus. Skip such high-fat choices as Gouda or Asiago cheese and spreads like olive and pine nut. Soups such as zesty lentil, chicken noodle, and chicken tortilla are filling yet easy on the calories. Red beans and rice or black bean soup is even healthier because it has more fiber.

Wrap places. Wrap sandwiches are popular, and sandwich shops everywhere offer them. They fill their wraps with grilled lean beef or chicken and lots of vegetables, like tomatoes, peppers, onions, and even roasted potatoes. Don't forget beans (everything from black beans to pinto beans).

Supermarkets. What could be faster than running in and grabbing a lunch-size salad in a bag, some string cheese, a box of crackers, and a couple pieces of fresh fruit? Other good ideas: dried fruit, bite-size cereal, and small cartons of milk or juice. If you need a bowl or plate, or even a plastic spoon or fork, head to the deli department and ask for one. They normally provide these items free of charge.

Fish and Seafood

Fish is almost all protein and keeps you satisfied for hours. Protein also "feeds" your blood sugar over 4 to 6 hours, rather than just an hour or so like carbs do. The result? Protein helps you eat less over the long haul. Also, it rebuilds muscle and powers the millions of chemical reactions that sustain you during body-shaping workouts.

Compared with other sources of protein, like meat or cheese, fish is relatively lean—from 2 to 8 percent fat, depending on the species. (In comparison, a well-marbled porterhouse steak weighs in at 48 percent fat.) The trouble arises when fish comes gift-wrapped in batter, butter, or other high-calorie coatings.

Shopping Smarts

While fresh fish certainly remains the most delectable way to enjoy fish, there are now several convenient ways to make including fish in your diet easier. Fortunately, options are now available in frozen and "convenience" fish, beyond the breaded and fried fillets or oily canned selections that quickly negate the reason you've chosen fish.

Canned fish. If you're an old hand at the diet game, you already know that 3 ounces of water-packed tuna has 53 fewer calories and 5.3 grams of fat less than oil-packed tuna. If you'd welcome a little variety in your fish repertoire, try tuna's cold-water cousins-in-a-can: salmon, clams, sardines, and anchovies. Look for water-packed versions of salmon, sardines, and clams. If you like anchovies, save them for special occasions. They supply as many as 180 calories and 12 grams of fat in 3 ounces.

As for tuna salad, if you make it at home with fat-free mayo, you're in the clear. Tuna salads from the supermarket deli case, though, are pretty heavy on the regular mayonnaise.

Frozen fish. Time was, your choices were pretty much limited to "white bread" varieties like haddock, cod, flounder, and halibut. Today supermarkets offer a virtual smorgasbord of fish. In addition to the old standards, you can find just about any finfish that's fit to eat—swordfish, perch, orange roughy, monkfish, snapper, catfish. Throw a couple of fillets on the grill with some lemon and herbs and you've added zero fat and calories but a whole lot of zip in just minutes. Or whip up a fish stew or chowder with fat-free milk. Serve with a salad and oyster crackers and it's chow time.

The Best Fish and Seafood

Fatty fish like salmon, tuna, and swordfish have slightly more fat and calories than white fish like haddock and cod. But those calories are worthwhile—they supply omega-3 fatty acids, which are beneficial to heart health.

Whether you're cooking fish at home or ordering it out, the key is to keep to a minimum the added fat and calories from butter and cream sauces, limiting the total calories from any fish entrée to 150 and the grams of fat to 5. The exception: casseroles containing fish, where you need to allow for calories from rice, noodles, milk, or other added components of the dish.

Entrée	Portion	Calories	Grams of Fat
Steamed crabmeat	3 oz	87	1.5
Haddock (broiled or baked)	3 oz	95	0.8
Albacore tuna packed in water	3 oz	105	1.5
Steamed shrimp with 2 Tbsp cocktail sauce	3 oz	114	0.9
Tuna (broiled or grilled)	3 oz	118	1.0
Broiled lobster tail with lemon juice	6 oz	166	1.0

If you can afford it, help yourself to shrimp, lobster, or crab. Although these crustaceans are higher in cholesterol than most other types of fish, studies have shown that eating shrimp, for example, lowers triglyceride levels and raises high-density lipoprotein (the good variety) cholesterol levels. Ten large steamed or broiled shrimp have just 54 calories and barely 0.5 gram of fat. If it is consumed without butter, even lobster is totally figure-friendly.

"Imitation" fish. Check the frozen fish case for fully cooked, packaged fish labeled as imitation crab, imitation lobster, and imitation scallops. Commonly made from white fish, they are exceptionally low in fat; in fact, most varieties are fat-free. Just open a package and top your salad with a generous 3 ounces of imitation crabmeat chunks. You'll reel in just 87 calories, 10 grams of protein—and only 1 gram of fat. For a quick entrée, combine packaged fish with a bag of frozen vegetables in a stir-fry. If you're allergic to shellfish, always read the label to make sure the brand you've chosen doesn't include any of the real stuff for flavor, as some do.

Gravies and Sauces

Good gravy, girlfriend! What's that on your mashed potatoes? Isn't gravy one of the biggest dieting no-nos there is? Well . . . not necessarily. True, good old-fashioned home-style gravy made with a mess of meat drippings isn't such a hot idea. The calories and fat in it add up mighty fast. But lighter versions are now available—and that goes for many of our other favorite fatty sauces as well.

Before you take that as license to smother everything you eat in silken sauces, remember that many foods taste fine without embellishment. By preparing meat, poultry, fish, and vegetables in ways that preserve their natural flavors, you do away with the need to gussy them up. But for those times when something extra is called for, follow this advice.

Shopping Smarts

In addition to looking for lighter versions of your sauce favorites, think of entirely new ways to jazz up the plain meat, vegetables, or even dessert on your plate. Then go to the market with these tips in mind.

Gravies. The major manufacturers offer all sorts of nonfat gravies. In addition to regular beef, pork, chicken, and turkey gravy, you'll find mushroom, zesty onion, au jus, slow-roasted types, rotisserie flavors, and more. Even the ones that aren't fat-free typically have only a gram or two of fat per ¼-cup serving.

The flavor is surprisingly good, although they may be a little on the salty side. If the texture is too thick for your taste, thin the gravy with water, broth, or wine when you heat it.

Creamy sauces. Béarnaise and hollandaise are diet busters. A typical béarnaise sauce has 12 grams of fat in just 2 tablespoons. Hollandaise can run about that much, too. If it's creaminess you're after, try reduced-fat condensed soups. Thinned-down cream of chicken, mushroom, celery, and broccoli make good toppings for simply prepared chicken, fish, and rice. Horseradish stirred into fat-free mayonnaise, yogurt, or sour cream makes a superb sauce for roast beef. Replace the horseradish with dill for fish, shrimp, and other seafood. An envelope of dry salad dressing, such as ranch or roasted garlic, combined with 2 cups of fat-free sour cream and a little milk is good on baked or mashed potatoes.

Salsas. They perk up everything from fish fillets and chicken breast to meat loaf and baked potatoes. There are literally dozens of varieties available, including green ones made from cactus or tomatillos. Most are nearly fat-free; check the label to be sure.

Other savory sauces. Make leftover vegetables work for you. Puree cooked red peppers, broccoli, or carrots with broth or wine. Start with 1 cup of vegetables and 1 tablespoon of broth or wine. Add more liquid if you want a thinner sauce or more vegetables if you want a thicker one. Add the seasonings of your choice. The sauce can be used as a topping for meat, poultry, or seafood. Or try defatted broth as a light, refreshing glaze for meat or poultry. Simply boil it in a saucepan until it's reduced to half or less of its original volume. (Use reduced-sodium broth to keep the glaze from becoming too salty.)

The Best Gravies and Sauces

If you're sizing up a sauce or gravy, those with fewer than 110 calories and less than 3 grams of fat are decent choices. Even meat gravy can make the grade—provided you don't empty the whole gravy boat over your plate.

Gravy or Sauce	Portion	Calories	Grams of Fat
Tomato sauce	¼ cup	18	0.2
Fat-free gravy	¼ cup	20	0.0
Au jus gravy	¼ cup	24	0.3
Reduced-fat cream of mushroom soup	¼ cup	35	1.5
Regular meat gravy	2 Tbsp	40	3.0
Horseradish sauce made with nonfat mayonnaise	2 Tbsp	44	0.9
Raspberry sauce	¼ cup	50	0.3
Nonfat caramel sauce	2 Tbsp	100	0.0
Cranberry sauce	¼ cup	100	0.1
Nonfat chocolate sauce	2 Tbsp	110	0.0

Tomato sauce is good for more than just pasta. Chicken breasts, fish fillets, and baked potatoes taste great with a tomato sauce topping. Look for ones with 2 grams or less of fat per ½-cup serving. As for pesto sauce, be careful. Even the reduced-fat type isn't what you'd call low in fat. Just 2 tablespoons have 15 grams of fat. The good thing about pesto is its assertive flavor—a little goes a long way. Thin it with defatted broth, or stir a spoonful into nonfat sour cream, yogurt, or pureed cottage cheese. Then serve it with poultry, seafood, steamed vegetables, and baked potatoes.

Dessert sauces. Forget about custard sauce when serving angel food cake, reduced-fat pound cake, poached pears, and other desserts. Instead, try nonfat chocolate, vanilla, or butterscotch pudding (make it thinner by using an extra ½ cup of milk when you cook it). Or go with flavored yogurt (add a little grated orange rind to kick up the flavor). You might also want to try sweetening fat-free sour cream or plain yogurt with brown sugar. Don't overlook cranberry sauce (try orange- or raspberry-flavored), chunky applesauce, crushed pineapple, and pureed raspberries or strawberries. Also consider fat-free butterscotch, caramel, and chocolate sauces for ice cream and frozen yogurt.

Weight-Friendly Substitutions

Turn your back on unwanted calories with these saucy stand-ins.

- Knock off calories in creamy sauces by substituting evaporated skim milk for cream. Another idea: For every cup of cream sauce, slowly whisk 1 tablespoon of flour into 1 cup of cold fat-free milk until smooth, then stir over medium heat until the mixture comes to a boil. Continue to stir for a minute or two to get rid of the raw-flour taste. Season with salt and pepper plus your choice of herbs, mustard, Parmesan cheese, shredded low-fat cheese, or horseradish. You can use the same technique with defatted broth or a combination of broth and milk.

- For glossy, somewhat transparent sauces, substitute cornstarch for the flour, but use ½ tablespoon of cornstarch for every tablespoon of flour in the original recipe.
- Prepare your favorite packaged sauce mixes with fat-free milk and half the butter or margarine.
- When making gravy, degrease the meat or poultry juices with a fat-separating pitcher before continuing with the recipe. Thicken the juices with either flour or cornstarch first dissolved in a little cold water.
- Instead of adorning vegetables with cheese sauce, toss them with lemon juice, fat-free Italian dressing, or a dash of hot sauce.

New Foods to Try

You may think it impossible to cut back on gravy and savory sauces. But other flavor enhancers can take their place. Flavored vinegars, such as tarragon and raspberry, add zest without fat. So do mustards, such as honey, peppercorn, and Dijon. They go great with meat. If they're not "saucelike" enough for you, mix them with nonfat sour cream. For more ideas, see "Condiments and Spreads," on page 52.

Meat

Got a beef with beef? Well, lighten up! Beef has. So have other meats like pork, lamb, and veal. If you've been eating poultry and fish every night in the name of slimming down, you can stop now. Leaner cuts abound in the meat case, and they add up to calorie savings. For example, seven cuts of beef and eight cuts of pork have a little more fat than skinless chicken breast, but less than skinless chicken thighs.

Giving up meat can, in fact, be a person's downfall. Meat supplies the nutrients busy people need to keep going. Three ounces of cooked meat provides about 50 percent of the Daily Value for protein, approximately 25 percent of the zinc and niacin, and up to about 17 percent of the iron.

Balance, variety, and moderation are the cornerstones of a nutritious eating plan you can stick with in the long run. That includes modest portions of beef, pork, veal, lamb, ham, and even lunchmeat. Most women need only about 6 ounces of meat, chicken, or seafood a day. Three ounces of lean meat a few times a week will do you more good than harm.

Shopping Smarts

When shopping for meat, think, "Buy less, eat less." Start by keeping high-fat meats out of your shopping cart and concentrating on leaner versions. If you get a good buy on lean meat, use a small amount now and freeze the extra in 3-ounce portions. That's about the size of a deck of cards. Here are the best buys at the meat counter.

Beef. Find out whether the beef your market sells is graded prime, choice, or select. Prime has the most fat marbled throughout; select has the least. Choose cuts with the word *loin* or *round* in the name for the fewest calories and the least fat. Eye of round, top round, round tip, top sirloin, bottom round, top loin, and tenderloin are the lowest-fat choices. When selecting ground beef, go for the highest percentage of lean that you can find. Ground top round (97 percent lean) and ground sirloin (90 percent) are the best choices.

Pork. The leanest cuts are tenderloin, sirloin chops, loin roast, top loin chops, loin chops, sirloin roast, rib chops, and rib roast. Check your market for Smithfield Lean Generation Pork, which is specially bred to be low in fat. Despite its reputation, ham is also lean, as long as the exterior fat has been trimmed off. Bacon? Regular, no. Canadian bacon, yes—it's made from cured pork loin.

Veal. The cuts that are lowest in fat include arm, blade, steak, rib roast, loin chops, and cutlets. Cook veal in ways that keep it lean—that means not making a habit of veal cordon bleu (veal stuffed with ham and cheese) or veal Oscar (veal topped with crab and buttery béarnaise sauce).

Lamb. Look for arm chops, loin chops, shank, and leg roast. Grill the chops, braise the shank, and make vegetable-rich stew with the leg meat.

The Best Meat Selections

It's generally a good idea to zero in on cuts or entrées with fewer than 350 calories and less than 9 grams of fat per serving. But of the two, fat content is a better benchmark. For example, bacon doesn't have a lot of calories, but most of those calories come from fat, not protein.

Meat	Portion	Calories	Grams of Fat
Lean roast beef from deli	3 slices (3 oz)	120	4.5
Canadian bacon	3 slices (3 oz)	129	5.8
Pork tenderloin	3 oz	139	4.1
Roasted beef eye of round	3 oz	141	4.0
Beef top round	3 oz	169	4.3
Flank steak	3 oz	176	8.6
Broiled pork sirloin chops	3 oz	181	8.6
Lamb shish kebabs	3 oz	190	7.5
Beef and broccoli stir-fry	4 oz	346	3.9

Weight-Friendly Substitutions

Even when you're using lean meat, don't get carried away. Make a habit of cutting the amount you use by trying protein-rich substitutes, like the following.

- Use marinated firm tofu in traditional meat and vegetable stir-fries. Serve over rice.
- Make tacos and burritos with only half the meat. Toss in rinsed canned beans to make up the difference. Likewise, prepare your favorite chili recipe with half meat and half beans.
- Substitute the following for 1 ounce of meat: one large egg, ¼ cup egg substitute, 1 ounce chicken or turkey, 1 ounce seafood, ½ cup cooked dried beans (including lentils and split peas), ¼ cup fat-free or low-fat cottage cheese (2 ounces), 8 ounces fat-free or low-fat yogurt, or 1 ounce of tofu, tempeh, or textured vegetable protein.
- Use your slow cooker to make meat and vegetable meals. The long, slow cooking time tenderizes lean cuts of meat.
- Substitute rice for half the meat in stuffed peppers.
- Replace some of the ground beef in pasta sauces and meat pies with ground turkey breast.

New Foods to Try

Feeling adventurous? Consider game meats. Venison, elk, bison, and rabbit are exceptionally lean. Venison, elk, and bison may be made as pot roasts or as chops, and rabbit is tasty braised. If you're timid about trying them "straight up," use them in mixed dishes such as stews and tacos.

Soybean products, such as tofu and tempeh, have gone mainstream and are good replacements for some of the meat in recipes. Try them in stir-fries, chili, and pasta sauces. The same goes for textured vegetable protein crumbles, which mimic ground meat in shape and protein content.

Milk and Dairy

For women, milk and dairy foods supply hefty amounts of calcium, much needed for strong bones, plus decent amounts of muscle-building protein and the essential vitamins B_{12} and riboflavin. As a bonus, milk is fortified with vitamin D, which offers added bone protection.

If you're not careful, however, milk, like all animal foods, can serve up fair amounts of fat and calories with the valuable vitamins and minerals it supplies. And if you have trouble digesting lactose, the sugar naturally found in milk, you can end up with bloating, abdominal cramps, gas, or diarrhea. Below, you'll find out how to sidestep both problems so that you can make milk a part of your eating-lean plan. (For information on cheese, see page 45.)

Shopping Smarts

If you're watching your weight, you're probably already buying fat-free or reduced-fat milk. With 8.1 grams of fat and 150 calories per cup, whole milk gives you almost as many calories and fat as a handful of potato chips. Instead, look for:

Reduced-fat milk. At 4.7 grams of fat and 121 calories per cup, 2 percent milk (reduced-fat) is a great intermediate step in coming down from whole milk to fat-free. Switching to fat-free can help you shed the pounds that shave off inches effortlessly. If you drink three glasses of milk daily, switching from 2 percent to fat-free milk will help you shed a pound every month or so. Note that skim milk is now called fat-free milk or nonfat milk on labels.

If you've avoided fat-free milk in the past because it tasted watery to you, look for protein-fortified products—the extra protein gives them the rich body of whole or reduced-fat milk, with less fat and fewer calories.

Fat-free evaporated milk. Does your pumpkin pie recipe call for evaporated milk? Substitute the fat-free variety—the only thing you'll miss is the calories. Fat-free evaporated milk works in cream sauces, too, saving loads of calories.

Coffee creamer. Creamers do contain fat. If you drink coffee on a regular basis, you're better off using milk. Suppose you normally use 1 tablespoon of nondairy powdered

The Best Milk and Dairy Selections

As a rule, look for milk that contains no fat and 85 calories per 8 ounces, coffee creamer that offers 1.5 grams of fat and 45 calories per tablespoon, sour cream and cream cheese that contain no fat and 14 calories per tablespoon, yogurt that contains no fat and 100 calories per 8 ounces, and fat-free frozen yogurt and ice cream that contain no fat and 140 calories per ½-cup serving.

Food Item	Portion	Calories	Grams of Fat
Fat-free milk	1 cup	85	0.4
Low-fat buttermilk	1 cup	99	2.2
Sherbet	½ cup	102	1.5
Low-fat milk	1 cup	102	2.6
Unsweetened fat-free yogurt	1 cup	137	0.4
Soy milk	1 cup	141	2.8
Low-fat chocolate milk	1 cup	158	2.5

creamer in your coffee daily, and you drink two cups of coffee a day. If you switch to 2 tablespoons of reduced-fat milk instead, you'll drop a pound effortlessly in about 7 weeks.

Or look for fat-free flavored coffee creamers, such as café mocha, Irish cream, and amaretto.

Sour cream. At 2.5 grams of fat and 28 calories per tablespoon, sour cream isn't so bad provided that you limit how much you use. By substituting the lower-fat version, you can either use more or save calories. Making guacamole or sour cream dip? Use reduced-fat sour cream (1.8 grams of fat and 20 calories per tablespoon) or nonfat sour cream (zero gram of fat and 13 calories per tablespoon). Switching from regular sour cream to nonfat practically slashes calories in half and wipes out a whopping 5 grams of fat in 2 tablespoons—the amount most people use on a baked potato.

Stretch sour cream by mixing 1 tablespoon of the low-fat or the full-fat version with salsa. On baked potatoes, try sour cream with picante tomato salsa. On fish, try sour cream with fruit salsa. Or add finely chopped onions and bell peppers.

Cream cheese. A tablespoon of regular cream cheese has 5 grams of fat and 51 calories. In comparison, fat-free cream cheese harbors a mere trace of fat and 14 calories. (Light, or low-fat, cream cheese supplies 2.5 grams of fat and 35 calories.) If you have a hard time making the switch to fat-free, buy the low-fat and fat-free versions and mix them, creating a version with 1.4 grams of fat and 25 calories. As your tastebuds adjust over time, you'll be able to make the switch all the way down to the fat-free version.

You might also want to try fruit- or herb-flavored low-fat versions, like raspberry- or strawberry-flavored cream cheese.

Yogurt. The choices are mind-boggling: full-fat, reduced-fat, fat-free. With fruit or fruit syrup—or plain.

With sugar or with artificial sweetener. Along with those choices comes a range of fat and calorie totals, from 3 grams of fat and 230 calories for full-fat, naturally sweetened yogurt to as little as zero gram of fat and 100 calories for the fat-free, artificially sweetened variety. Still, scouting out yogurt you like is worth the effort: For busy women, a container of yogurt makes an instant power-packed mini-meal or snack.

To select yogurt, start by homing in on products that are fat-free. Then check out the calories. Choose a product with no more than 120 calories in 8 ounces or 100 calories in 6 ounces. Or look for plain, vanilla, or lemon nonfat yogurt and slice your own fruit into the container.

Frozen yogurt and ice cream. Saving up calories for a daily dessert helps you stay on the lean eating track. It takes only about 150 calories to satisfy this desire for pleasurable food—just the amount in appropriately chosen frozen yogurt or ice cream. Choosing well means not only ferreting out the best calorie bargain but also the rich flavor that still satisfies in a controlled portion. Experiment with flavors that interest you, such as black raspberry swirl nonfat frozen yogurt or caramel-praline crunch nonfat frozen yogurt. Limit your serving to a ½ cup.

As for real ice cream, save it for topping the occasional hot low-fat fruit compote or crisp. Use only a ¼ cup and enjoy every rich bite slowly.

Digestion-Friendly Substitutions

Milk sugar, or lactose, is made up of two other sugars, glucose and galactose. The intestinal tract releases an enzyme, called lactase, to break apart the milk sugar; it then sends the sugar subunits through the rest of the metabolic pathway. When this works well, you don't even know it's happening. But when a person doesn't produce enough lactase, however, she is often miserable, suffering from abdominal gas and sometimes diarrhea. Fortunately, there are several options for lactose-intolerant people.

- Buy lactase-treated milk, such as Lactaid and DairyEase 100. Like other milks, it comes in a range of varieties, from full-fat to fat-free, so ferret out that nonfat or fat-free label.
- Purchase untreated milk and add lactase enzyme drops (available at drug stores).
- Take a lactase enzyme in pill form (also sold in drugstores) before eating or drinking anything containing milk. Follow the label directions.
- Try soy milk, which is naturally lactose-free. Soy milk's taste has improved dramatically over the years. To get the most bone-building power from soy milk, choose a variety that has been fortified with calcium, vitamin D, and vitamin B_{12}. Look for low-fat versions. (Fat-free soy milk isn't widely available.)
- If you're having a little trouble after taking antibiotics, the antibiotics may have upset the natural balance of bacteria in your intestinal tract. If so, try acidophilus milk, which is fortified with *Lactobacillus acidophilus* bacteria, thought to restore nature's balance in the intestinal tract. Choose the 1 percent fat version. Low-fat buttermilk also works well to restore healthy bacteria in the gut.
- Buy calcium-fortified orange juice if you don't or can't drink milk.

New Foods to Try

Your options go beyond plain milk. Consider:

Yogurt cheese. Looking for something very low in fat and unique in flavor to spread on your toast or bagel?

Spread a coffee filter into a metal strainer and pour in a pint container of nonfat plain, vanilla, or lemon yogurt. Place the strainer in a bowl, cover, and place in the refrigerator overnight. In the morning, you'll find a thick, rich "cheese" that you can spread on breakfast bread. Stir in herbs, chopped veggies, diced fruit—or any combination of these—for a fat-free party spread.

Chocolate milk. Want something chocolate right now? Keep a quart of low-fat chocolate milk in the refrigerator and next to it a chilled 8-ounce glass. When a chocolate craving strikes, you can pour yourself half a glass (4 ounces) of chocolate milk and no more, using up just 79 calories.

Pasta and Toppings

Pasta is filling, low in fat, packed with energy-producing complex carbohydrates, and generally cholesterol-free. It's also a good source of B vitamins. You can't go wrong with all that nutrition for about 200 calories per serving. Where you *can* go wrong is topping your tagliatelle with fatty Alfredo, carbonara, pesto, or sausage or other meat sauces.

Shopping Smarts

Happily, you don't have to give pasta the boot when cutting calories. Just keep these things in mind when shopping.

Pasta. With so many shapes and sizes available, you can have pasta every night for weeks without ever repeating a meal. Buy strands like spaghetti and fettuccine, tubes like penne and ziti, various colored spirals, and shells of all sizes. Don't forget lasagna noodles and elbow macaroni for casseroles, cannelloni and manicotti for stuffing, and small shapes like orzo, stars, and acini di peppe for soups.

Check labels carefully when buying fresh pasta, especially stuffed types like ravioli, cappelletti, and tortellini.

Fresh pasta often contains eggs and is generally higher in fat than dried. In addition, the fillings in stuffed varieties are usually high in fat.

Sauce. Stick with low-fat, meatless tomato sauces rather than creamy ones like Alfredo and pesto. Even reduced-fat pesto can have 4 grams of fat in just 1 tablespoon. Look for sauces with 4 grams or less of fat per ½-cup serving. Be especially vigilant when reading labels for creamy sauces. Often the serving size has been reduced to ¼ cup—less than you might actually use.

The Best Pasta and Toppings

When you're planning a pasta meal, aim for about 300 calories per serving and 4 grams of fat or less (although you can afford a few more calories if the fat content is much lower).

Pasta or Topping	Portion	Calories	Grams of Fat
Sapsago cheese	1 oz (2 Tbsp)	16	0.5
Parmesan cheese	1 Tbsp	23	1.5
Pasta	1 cup cooked	197	1.0
Pasta primavera (with garlic and oil, not a cream-based sauce)	About 3 Tbsp sauce over 1 cup cooked pasta	239	4.5
Linguini with red clam sauce	½ cup sauce over 1 cup cooked pasta	257	2.0
Pasta with clam sauce (water, clams, oil, and spices)	¼ cup sauce over 1 cup cooked pasta	267	6.0
Pasta with marinara sauce	½ cup sauce over 1 cup cooked pasta	268	2.6

Pasta-ready tomatoes are also a good choice and are very low in fat. Look for flavors other than Italian for a change of pace. Taco-style Mexican sauce can give your pasta a whole new identity.

Cheese. If it's just not Italian without a dusting of cheese, make it a really flavorful type. Packaged grated Parmesan and Romano are okay in a pinch—there are even some reduced-fat varieties. But freshly grated or shredded cheese has far more flavor, so you can actually use less and still get great taste. Buy a thin wedge of really good cheese (like Parmigiano-Reggiano or Pecorino Romano) and grate it at the table. Tightly wrapped, it will keep in the refrigerator or freezer for weeks, so you can always have some on hand. Almost as flavorful is Parmesan or Romano that has already been shredded; buy it in small quantities.

An interesting alternative to Parmesan is sapsago, a very hard cone-shaped cheese from Switzerland that's low in fat. It has a light green color and a pungent herbal flavor that adds unexpected punch to pasta.

Weight-Friendly Substitutions
Here's how to cut fat in some of your favorite pasta recipes.

- Replace ground beef in pasta sauces with ground turkey breast. You'll save about 65 calories per 3-ounce portion of meat.
- Let steamed mushrooms, onions, and bell peppers stand in for some of the meat in pasta sauce.
- For an awesome Alfredo sauce, substitute low-fat cottage cheese or ricotta cheese blended with milk for the cream in a traditional recipe.
- Slim down pesto sauce by substituting chicken broth for some of the oil and using fewer nuts and less cheese. Or dilute purchased reduced-fat pesto sauce with

chicken broth. Whatever method you choose, use pesto sauce sparingly since it will never be truly low-fat.

- Make homemade macaroni and cheese with fat-free milk and reduced-fat sharp Cheddar cheese. Add chopped cooked vegetables for extra fiber.
- Whip up pasta salads with fat-free Italian dressing instead of mayonnaise. Add canned, packed-in-water tuna and chopped vegetables for a meal in a dish.

New Foods to Try

Try whole wheat and spinach pastas. They contain up to three times the fiber of regular pasta. All sorts of other colors and flavors are available—including squid ink, beet, and garlic herb. The tastier the pasta itself, the less sauce you need. And don't forget the non-Italian types of noodles, like Japanese soba (made from buckwheat flour), udon (made from wheat or cornmeal), somen and ramen (made from wheat), rice, mung bean, and others.

Pizza and Toppings

Pizza is a nutritional powerhouse. The crust contains B vitamins and complex carbohydrates for energy. The tomato sauce supplies carbohydrates, vitamin C, lycopene (a natural substance that appears to protect against cancer), and little fat. The cheese provides protein as well as much-needed calcium to strengthen your bones. Topped off with vegetables, pizza serves as a meal in itself, providing fiber and vitamin A. For added protein, you can add lean meat or seafood. What more could a busy woman want?

A lot less fat. Fat is pizza's pitfall. That doesn't rule it out of your eating plan, however. With a bit of nutrition know-how, you can curtail pizza's calories and still satisfy yourself.

Shopping Smarts

It pays to purchase healthy pizza ingredients. That way, you can concoct a nutritious and satisfying meal on a moment's notice—and for a lot less than a pizzeria pie costs (in dollars *and* calories). Here's what to buy.

Crust. Look in the refrigerated case for prepared pizza crust. There are ready-formed ones and those in a tube. Either way, check labels to find the lowest in fat. Sometimes plain crusts are also available in the freezer section. Don't forget the box mixes; prepare them with less oil than is called for in the recipe.

Sauce. There are lots of low-fat pizza and pasta sauces to choose from. Look for ones with 4 grams or less of fat per ½ cup. Try different flavors to give your pizza extra sparkle.

The Best Pizza and Toppings

Your best bets give you fewer than 300 calories and less than 12 grams of fat per slice, including the topping.

Pizza	Portion	Calories	Grams of Fat
Thin-crust cheese pizza with peppers, mushrooms, and onions (fast-food)	1 slice (⅛ of pie)	190	8.0
Homemade pizza (with low-fat prepared pizza shell, fat-free sauce, 8 oz part-skim mozzarella cheese, and 1 cup steamed vegetables)	1 slice (⅙ of pie)	211	3.1
Thin-crust cheese pizza (fast-food)	1 slice (⅛ of pie)	225	10.0
Thin-crust cheese pizza with 1 oz Canadian bacon	1 slice (⅛ of pie)	268	12.0

Cheese. Pick up reduced-fat shredded cheeses. Mozzarella is standard, but it needn't be your only choice. There are good Italian and Mexican cheese blends, for instance, that make terrific pizza. Limit cheese to 8 ounces per large pizza. If there's a really flavorful full-fat hard cheese you love, such as sharp Cheddar, go ahead and get it. Just use less. (Other assertive, nontraditional cheeses to try include Asiago, feta, and blue.)

Other toppings. Favor veggies like onions, bell peppers, mushrooms, and pickled hot peppers—even a few olives, if you like. Buy super-lean ground beef or ground turkey breast. They're better meat choices than pepperoni, sausage, meatballs, and salami. Brown the ground meat in a nonstick skillet and drain it well before sprinkling it over the crust. Canadian bacon and lean ham are good replacements for regular bacon.

If you'll be making the pizza soon after you shop, stop at the supermarket's salad bar to pick up already sliced onions, peppers, mushrooms, and other fresh vegetables to top your pizza.

Frozen pizza. Steer clear of frozen deep-dish pizza; the fat is out of sight. If you must purchase frozen pizza, pick a thin-crust variety. Enhance its nutrition by adding steamed or sautéed vegetables, lean ground beef, or diced cooked chicken. (Leftovers work great as pizza toppings.)

Here are other slimming substitutions.

- Sun-dried tomatoes can stand in for pepperoni. They have a similar look, but the intensely flavored tomatoes are much lower in fat. (Be sure to drain them of as much oil as possible.)
- Instead of sausage, try eggplant, portobello mushrooms, broccoli, jalapeño peppers, spinach, tomato slices, artichoke hearts, or zucchini. Pair drained

crushed pineapple or fresh pineapple pieces with lean ham, or have shrimp or clams instead of meat.

- Skip the cheese and pile on more vegetables to take up the slack. If it's calcium you're concerned about, have a glass of fat-free milk or a scoop of low-fat cottage cheese with your pizza.

- Select whole wheat crust whenever possible. It adds fiber and a nutty flavor to your pizza pie. Low-fat tortillas and pita rounds make great personal-size pizza crusts.

Potatoes and Toppings

Although one of America's favorite foods, spuds don't get the respect they deserve—from dieters or anyone else. The truth is that these tubers are tasty, versatile, convenient, and nutritious. But much like pasta, potatoes are often maligned because of the fattening company they keep.

That's too bad, because potatoes are a nutritional bargain. For about 150 calories, a baked white potato contributes complex carbohydrates and fiber, supplies more potassium than a medium banana, and provides one-third of the Daily Value for vitamin C. All that for zero fat and cholesterol. Sweet potatoes provide comparable nutrition, with a bonus: a bounty of beta-carotene—a powerful weapon in fighting off diseases like cancer.

It all boils down to this: In their freshest forms, white potatoes and sweet potatoes are innocent of all the fattening charges leveled against them. As long as you don't eat them too often in their high-fat versions—scalloped, au gratin, or fried, for example—potatoes can most certainly be part of your successful slimming plan.

Shopping Smarts
Whenever possible, use whole raw potatoes. Here's what to look for.

White potatoes. Look for spuds that are clean, firm, smooth, and regular in shape. Pass up any with wrinkles, sprouts, cracks, soft dark areas, or green spots. Pick a variety for different uses. Long whites are good all-purpose potatoes with a waxy texture. Round whites and reds are good for boiling. Russets are the perfect baking potatoes. Store your potatoes in a cool, dark, well-ventilated place, where they'll last for several weeks. Don't keep them in the fridge, and don't store them near onions or they'll go bad faster.

The Best Potatoes and Toppings

Aim for 180 calories per serving and less than 4 grams of fat, including the topping.

Potato	Portion	Calories	Grams of Fat
Boiled potatoes	1 cup	113	0.1
Oven-baked sweet potato wedges	4 oz	117	0.1
Mashed potatoes with fat-free milk	1 cup	124	0.2
Candied sweet potato wedges	3.75 oz	144	3.4
Medium plain baked potato	5.5 oz	145	0.2
Boiled red potatoes, skin on, tossed with 1 tsp margarine or butter	1 cup	149	4.1
Medium baked sweet potato topped with 1 tsp brown sugar	5.5 oz	156	0.2
Medium baked potato with 1 Tbsp light sour cream	5.5 oz	165	2.0

Sweet potatoes. These potatoes should be firm, with bright, uniformly colored skin. There are two main types: moist and dry. The moist ones have orange skin and flesh and are usually called yams. The dry sweet potatoes have yellowish-tan skin and yellow flesh that's crumbly when cooked. Store both kinds unwrapped in a cool, dry, dark place for up to a week. Because sweet potatoes are high in beta-carotene, they deserve weekly appearances on your table.

Processed products. Instant mashed potatoes, scalloped and au gratin potato mixes, and ready-to-cook hash browns are certainly convenient. If you prepare them without added butter or margarine, they're actually low in fat. Their main drawbacks are low fiber, high sodium, and no vitamin C. Think of them as stand-ins for when you don't have time to prepare fresh potatoes. Treat potato chips—even the fat-free ones—as just that: treats. They don't count as a vegetable!

Weight-Friendly Substitutions

Here's how to pep up potatoes without blowing your calorie budget.

- Top baked potatoes with 1 tablespoon of light sour cream instead of butter. Or sprinkle spuds with butter-flavored flakes.
- Mix plain nonfat yogurt, chopped cucumbers, dried dill, salt, and pepper for a terrific tuber topper. Other ideas: soy sauce and sesame seeds; sautéed mushrooms and onions; fat-free cottage cheese mixed with chives; salsa and nonfat sour cream.
- Opt for a medium baked potato with 1 tablespoon of low-fat sour cream instead of 20 french fries.
- Cube sweet and white potatoes and toss with a little olive oil. Roast at 400°F for about 20 minutes, or until tender.

- Make your own potato chips. Slice white or sweet potatoes into very thin rounds and toss with a drizzle of canola oil. Place in a single layer on a baking sheet and bake at 400°F until crispy, about 10 minutes.
- Use cubed sweet potatoes as a stand-in for some of the beef in traditional beef stew and soup recipes.
- Snack on sweet potatoes instead of potato chips or fries. Keep baked sweet potatoes in the refrigerator. Peel and slice for a sweet, fiber-packed snack or sandwich companion.

New Foods to Try

If you think Peruvian Purple, Yukon Gold, and Red Cloud are next fall's fashion colors, you haven't been hanging out in the produce aisle. They're names of potatoes you should try. Potatoes now come in wonderful new shades and shapes, so you can serve them often but not feel like you're eating the same thing all the time. Yukon Gold, Yellow Finn, and Daisy Gold are marked by moist yellow flesh that boasts a buttery flavor. They're great mashed, baked, or roasted. Look for other interesting types, like All-Blue, Purple Chief, Rose Finn Apple, and Russian Banana. "New" potatoes are simply spuds of any type picked small. They're excellent boiled or roasted whole.

Salad Dressings

Salads have great potential for being naturally low in fat and calories—if you stick to vegetables, fruits, grain products, and other lean or low-fat ingredients. After all, vegetables and fruits have little or no fat. Besides their nutrients, they can supply fair amounts of fiber, which fills you up without adding calories.

When it comes to "dressing up" a salad, though, you need to proceed carefully. In a study of women 19 to 50 years old, salad dressings were their primary source of dietary fat. Here's how to scout out figure-friendly dressings.

Shopping Smarts

The quickest way to put your salad on a diet is to stock up on bottled reduced-fat or fat-free dressings. If you have a few minutes, make your own fresh, more flavorful versions. To create a little salad magic on short notice, just keep on hand a variety of vinegars, oils, and seasonings as well as yogurt or low-fat buttermilk. Either way, here's what to look for.

The Best Salad Dressings

You can dress your salad without any fat by tossing it with a bit of lemon or pineapple juice or a dash of balsamic or flavored vinegar. Or look for salad dressings that have no more than 3 grams of fat and 40 calories per serving. Just be aware that the serving size listed on the label is often quite small, so carefully measure the amount you put on your salad.

Salad Dressing	Portion	Calories	Grams of Fat
Balsamic vinegar	1 Tbsp	10	0.0
Fat-free mayonnaise	1 Tbsp	10	0.0
Fat-free Italian	2 Tbsp	15	0.0
Low-fat mayonnaise	1 Tbsp	25	1.0
Fat-free French	2 Tbsp	30	0.0
Fat-free vinaigrette	2 Tbsp	35	0.0
Low-fat raspberry vinaigrette	2 Tbsp	35	1.5
Fat-free ranch	2 Tbsp	40	0.0
Low-fat blue cheese	2 Tbsp	40	1.5

Prepared salad dressings. Because manufacturers may use various starches and stabilizers as fat replacers, these dressings aren't entirely calorie-free. And with so much variety, the number of calories in these products varies. To find those with the fewest calories, check out the Nutrition Facts on the food label. Experiment to find which ones you like best.

You might also look for packaged salad dressing mixes at the store. Just add vinegar and oil, using less oil and more vinegar.

Vinegars. Vinegar has practically no calories and can be paired with any oil—in proportions you control—plus a number of savory herbs and flavorings. Start with the basics: cider vinegar, red wine vinegar, and white vinegar. Try dark, sweet balsamic vinegar for a unique, strong flavor that is great on greens. When you're following a recipe for an oil-and-vinegar vinaigrette, cut back on the oil and use more vinegar.

Oils. All oils have about the same amount of fat and calories—14 grams of fat and 125 calories per tablespoon. Olive oil is high in monounsaturated fat, which can actually help lower your total cholesterol count. Don't assume that "light" olive oil has fewer calories—it's simply lighter in flavor and color, not fat.

To get the most flavor from the least oil on salads, choose stronger-flavored oils, such as extra-virgin olive oil, sesame oil, walnut or other nut oils, or herb-infused oils.

Seasonings. Boost the flavor of homemade dressings with fresh herbs. Tarragon, oregano, basil, and parsley are basics. Keep fresh or minced, jarred garlic on hand, too.

Weight-Friendly Substitutions

Using low-fat dressing from your supermarket is one way to cut fat and calories. Here are others.

In place of high-fat dressings:

- Fill a spray bottle with a full-flavored oil to lightly spritz your greens. You'll end up using much less oil.
- Skip the oil entirely, and just dress your greens with balsamic vinegar. Or try an herb- or berry-flavored vinegar that you can buy at the store or make yourself.
- Toss salads with a splash of juice or a mixture of juices—orange, tangerine, lemon, lime, pineapple, and tomato juice all work well—and freshly ground pepper.
- For a creamy homemade dressing for tossed salad, slaw, potato salad, or chicken salad, use plain fat-free yogurt thinned with low-fat buttermilk. Add minced fresh herbs, such as chives, tarragon, or dill.
- Puree low-fat cottage cheese in a blender. Add fat-free milk or low-fat buttermilk and flavor with fresh herbs, Parmesan cheese, and pepper.

To dress up dressing:

- Toss any dressing with minced herbs (such as tarragon, sage, thyme, parsley, basil, chervil, chives, or garlic), curry, poppy or celery seed, or capers.
- Add a few teaspoons of plain or fruit yogurt to herbed vinegar for a creamy version of vinaigrette.
- Blend a flavorful mustard or horseradish into vinaigrette or thinned yogurt.

No-fat ways to dress a salad:

- Grate a little orange, lime, or lemon peel or some fresh ginger over fresh greens, fruit salad, and poultry or seafood salad.
- In garden salads, toss in some distinctively flavored greens, such as watercress, endive, arugula, radicchio, or frisée.

- For pasta or garden salads, toss in chopped sun-dried tomatoes or chopped hot chile peppers.
- Toss green salads with edible flowers (purchased in the produce department, not at the florist).

Snacks

There's a lot more to snack on than candy—and it's stuff your body will thank you for. Smart snacks pack valuable nutrients along with satisfaction and comfort: vitamins A and C, fiber, and more. For example, you can increase folate with nuts, calcium with frozen yogurt, and fiber with fig bars. Make the right choices, and you can really nibble those excess pounds away.

Shopping Smarts

To find nutrient-dense snacks, read more than just the information about fat and calories on the label. Look for fiber, calcium, iron, and other vitamins and minerals. Take Rice Krispie Treat Bars, for example. These convenient treats rack up only 90 calories and 2 grams of fat apiece, but their real benefit is their vitamin and mineral fortification. They offer far more nutrition than a doughnut or sugar cookies.

Consider the "crunch factor" when choosing snacks. Crunchy foods like baby carrots, apple slices, daikon radishes (which are milder than regular radishes), cucumbers, and pickles take longer to eat than soft snack cakes, for instance. And they tend to be satisfying, so you may eat less of them. Here are other noteworthy noshes.

Cereal bars. These tend to be a better choice than granola bars because they're lower in fat and higher in nutrients. Many 1-ounce granola bars contain 128 calories and 5.8 grams of fat, while many cereal bars might have 92 calories and zero gram of fat. What really sets them apart, though, is the fact that cereal bars are fortified with between 10 and 50 percent of your Daily Value for many vitamins and minerals.

String cheese. This mozzarella-like cheese offers a helping of calcium without a lot of fat—as long as you don't eat the whole package. Look for the kind that's portion-controlled in sticks of ¾ ounce.

Nuts. They're filled with fiber, iron, and all kinds of trace minerals and immunity-enhancing nutrients. Their biggest drawback, of course, is fat (even though it's heartsmart unsaturated fat). But if you learn to eat just a

The Best Snacks

Obviously, nutrient-dense, naturally fat-free vegetables and fruits are smart snacks anytime. Otherwise, try to choose crackers, cookies, and other snacks with no more than 3 grams of fat in a 100-calorie serving. The exceptions: soy nuts and yucca chips. As snack foods go, they're incredibly nutrient dense, redeeming their fat and calorie contents.

Snack Food	Portion	Calories	Grams of Fat
Tomato juice	½ cup	20	0.0
Baby carrots with 1 Tbsp fat-free ranch dip	5 carrots	45	0.0
Air-popped popcorn	3 cups	90	0.0
Cereal bar	1 bar	92	3.0
Baked tortilla chips	13 chips (1 oz)	110	1.0
Baked potato chips	11 chips (1 oz)	110	1.5
Yucca chips	15–16 chips (1 oz)	130	6.0
Roasted soy nuts	⅓ cup (1 oz)	150	7.0

handful to satisfy that snack urge, you can reap their nutritional benefits. Remember that 1 ounce is considered a serving, and that's roughly ¼ cup. Soy nuts are surprisingly low in fat compared with other nuts. One ounce has 7 grams of fat compared with 14 grams for peanuts. An even better idea: chestnuts. Five chestnuts have only 103 calories and 1 gram of fat.

Popcorn. Air-popped popcorn has only 30 calories and no fat in 1 cup. Microwave popcorn is a whole other animal. Eat a bag of it and you've put away 33 grams or more of fat—more than half your daily allowance. If you can't resist microwave popcorn, look for light or low-fat types. Even then, take a good look at the label. The entire bag contains roughly three servings.

Chips. Save half the calories and all the fat by eating fat-free potato chips. Low-fat tortilla chips have only 90 calories and 1 gram of fat in a serving.

Weight-Friendly Substitutions
Smart substitutions may just mean finding a new version of a favorite high-fat food: Baked fat-free chips instead of regular. Chocolate caramel popcorn cakes rather than caramels. Cinnamon streusel rice cakes instead of cinnamon streusel coffee cake. Oreo cereal in place of Oreo cookies (it's fortified with extra vitamins and minerals that the cookies don't have). Other smart swaps:

- Soy nut butter instead of peanut butter. It's lower in fat and contains cancer-fighting isoflavones.
- Vegetable cocktail, tomato, grapefruit, or orange juice instead of empty-calorie soda.
- Reduced-fat Chex Mix instead of high-fat nut mixes.

New Foods to Try
A snack can be defined any way you want. Think beyond chips, doughnuts, and candy bars.

Dried fruit. Try cranberries, blueberries, and orange-flavor prunes in addition to the old standbys dried apricots, peaches, and pears. They're naturally sweet and chock-full of fiber and vitamins.

Fresh fruit. Get out of the bananas-and-oranges rut. Try other fruits, like mangoes, papayas, ugli fruit (a tangerine-grapefruit hybrid from Jamaica), champagne grapes, figs, Asian pears, and interesting apple varieties like Fuji, Royal Gala, Jonagold, and Braeburn.

Soup. Choose canned and instant soups that are high in fiber, like black bean, minestrone, lentil, and split pea. Pop it into the microwave for an instant snack.

Cereal. It's not just breakfast food. And even when sugarcoated, it is much more nutrient dense than cake, candy, and cookies. Eat bite-size cereal right out of the box. You can even find convenient snack-size bags of cereal, like Post Snack-Abouts.

Soy power bars. Choose ones that remind you of a decadent treat, like GeniSoy Soy Protein Bars in peanut butter fudge or apple spice yogurt. They're not only extremely satisfying but also filled with protein, fiber, and lots of vitamins.

Cracker Jack. Sweet, crunchy caramel corn with only 120 calories and 2 grams of fat in a ½ cup!

Yucca chips. Made from a starchy tropical root vegetable, these crisp chips have more than twice the fiber of regular potato chips—as well as 40 percent less fat. Available in flavors like barbecue, garlic, cilantro, and picante 'n' cream cheese, they're a terrific snack.

Office Snacks
Your good intentions needn't be left at home when you head to work. Just take along portable snacks like the following.

Desk-drawer delights. Stock up on light microwave popcorn, low-fat crackers, rice cakes, low-fat cookies, dried fruit, soy nuts, or cereal bars.

For the office fridge. Keep a stash of yogurt, baby carrots, cut-up vegetables, salad in a bag with low-fat dressing, skim milk, low-fat chocolate milk, hummus, and low-fat cream cheese spreads. (Travel tip: These snacks work great in the car; pack them in an insulated bag or cooler with ice packs.)

Soups and Chowders

Soup can serve as the prelude to a nutritious meal—or as its centerpiece. And because soup is sipped, not chewed, it takes time to eat, which is a benefit for women who tend to overeat. Studies suggest that people who start their meals with soup eat less food and consume fewer calories than those who do not.

Soup is versatile and, depending on the ingredients, supplies various amounts of valuable nutrients. Vegetable soup can be loaded with vitamins A and C, folate, and potassium. Hearty soups made with rice, pasta, or other grains contribute complex carbohydrates. Chowders made with milk fortify your diet with calcium. Bean soups, such as split pea or lentil, are satisfying ways to add fiber to your menu.

To build your soup repertoire, know the lingo. *Broth* is low in fat if it's been skimmed. *Consommé* is simply concentrated broth. *Chowder* is a thick, chunky soup made with milk or cream or thickened with a flour-butter mixture. *Bisque* is a rich, thick soup typically made with butter and cream. (But don't worry—you can easily "de-fat" chowder and other rich, creamy homemade soups or shop for low-fat varieties.)

Shopping Smarts

If you're like most people, you probably rely on canned soups for fast "heat and eat" meals. Supermarket shelves are stocked with every variety of soup imaginable. Think beyond old standbys like tomato and chicken noodle. For further versatility, you can combine two prepared soups or fortify them with a variety of mix-ins.

Clear soups are usually lower in fat and calories than creamy soups. You'll also find low-fat and fat-free versions of cream of mushroom, cream of celery, and other higher-fat soups. Very often, the heartier the soup, the more nutrients you get.

Whether you make soup from scratch or buy prepared soups, these health-smart tips can help you stock a soup-ready kitchen.

Canned broth. Fat-free vegetable, beef, and chicken broths serve as the bases for all kinds of soups. If you're sodium sensitive, buy broth with the lowest sodium content. Or make your own broth without added salt, then chill it and skim off the fat.

The Best Soups

When selecting soups to buy or prepare, your best choices are low-fat versions with 3 grams of fat or less per serving.

Soup	Portion	Calories	Grams of Fat
Miso soup	1 cup	35	0.0
Gazpacho soup	1 cup	56	0.2
Vegetable soup	1 cup	90	2.0
Minestrone	1 cup	120	2.0
Bean soup, made without bacon	1 cup	130	0.5
Chicken soup, made with defatted broth	1 cup	160	3.0

Ready-to-eat soups or condensed soups. Ready-to-eat soups simply need to be heated. With condensed soup, some of the water is removed, so you need to reconstitute them before heating. For more flavor and nutrients, use milk, broth, vegetable juice, or water left over from cooking vegetables, instead of plain water.

Dehydrated soups. Most are low in fat. To prepare, just add hot liquid, perhaps low-sodium broth.

Soup Up Your Soup

With a little creativity and a few simple items from the supermarket, you can add homemade flavor and a nutritional boost to low-fat soups. Here's what to look for.

- Canned stewed Mexican-flavored tomatoes, diced tomatoes flavored with Italian herbs, or plain, diced tomatoes. Add to corn chowder for a chunky texture.
- Pre-cut veggies (frozen, canned, or fresh, including stir-fry medleys) or cooked leftovers. Add to potato soup or other extra-chunky soups.
- Canned beans, such as black, cannellini (white kidney), kidney (red), or chickpeas. To reduce the sodium content, rinse the beans under running water before adding them to the soup. Mix them into vegetable noodle soup.
- Firm tofu. Slice and add to chicken noodle or vegetable soup.
- Canned crabmeat, clams, or diced chicken. Add to tomato soup.
- Tortellini, Chinese noodles, no-yolk egg noodles, or small pasta shapes, such as orzo, pastina, and couscous. These are especially good in turkey vegetable soup.
- Brown rice or barley. Mix into reduced-fat cream of mushroom soup.
- Sun-dried tomatoes or dried or canned mushrooms. Try them in onion or bean soup.

- From your freezer: Diced cooked skinless poultry, lean ground beef, seafood, leftover cooked meat, soy patties (to crumble for soup). Add them to vegetable soup for a hearty main dish.

Weight-Friendly Substitutions

If you're trying to slim down, you don't have to throw out your family's favorite recipes for chowder, potato, or other creamy soups or thick stews. You can lower the fat and boost the nutrients with these simple tricks.

Cream-based soup:

- Replace the cream with fat-free evaporated milk, low-fat buttermilk, or low-fat milk fortified with fat-free dry milk.
- For cold fruit soups, blend in fat-free yogurt (plain or fruit).

Thick, hearty soup or stew:

- Add starchy, raw vegetables, such as grated potatoes, yams, or parsnips. Simmer until thickened. In a hurry? Mix in potato flakes or leftover mashed potatoes instead. When the vegetables in your soup are thoroughly cooked, puree half, then stir the puree into the soup. (One cup of pureed vegetables thickens 3 to 4 cups of broth.)
- Blend in a small can of tomato paste.
- Simmer vegetable, chicken, or beef soup with rice, barley, oatmeal, or pasta, or try adding cooked, mashed beans.

Tacos, Tortilla Fillings, and Wraps

A taco is any rolled and stuffed corn tortilla, whether it's soft or crisp. As a handheld wrapping for various fillings, tortillas are just another form of sandwich bread. The basic difference is the flour—corn or wheat. Corn tortillas are somewhat lower in calories and fat. An 8-inch soft corn tortilla has about 1 gram of fat and 70 calories, compared with slightly more than 3 grams of fat and 115 calories in an 8-inch wheat tortilla. Taco shells are another story: They're fried to a crisp; two 5-inch shells carry about 6 grams of fat and 120 calories.

If you're making your own tortilla dishes, you can control calories and fat by tucking in plenty of vegetables; lean meat, poultry, and fish; and even fruit. You can also make filling mixtures with beans and rice. And tortillas can be moistened with salsas and other low-fat sauces and spreads.

The Best Tacos, Tortilla Fillings, and Wraps

Soft tortillas are generally lower in fat than taco shells, which are fried to make them crisp. Oven-baked tortilla chips have less fat than regular tortilla chips, too. For the stuffings, you can concoct a hearty filling with all kinds of low-fat and fat-free ingredients. Read the labels to compare.

Item, filling, or topping	Portion	Calories	Grams of Fat
Salsa	2 Tbsp	10	0.0
Fat-free sour cream	2 Tbsp	20	0.0
Corn tortilla	1 tortilla (1 oz)	70	0.6
Fat-free refried beans	½ cup	100	0.0
Baked tortilla chips	13 chips (1 oz)	110	1.0
Flour tortilla	1 tortilla (1¼ oz)	115	3.4

Whether you prefer Tex-Mex flavors or want to take your tastebuds beyond the border, here's how to fit tortillas and wraps into a weight-conscious eating plan for breakfast, lunch, dinner, and snacks.

Shopping Smarts

Wrap up quick, nutrition-minded meals today—starting with the tortillas, wraps, fillings, sauces, and seasonings you buy.

Tortillas. You can buy soft wheat and corn tortillas in various sizes, keep them on hand in your refrigerator or freezer, and use them when time for dinner is short. The 8- and 10-inch tortillas are fine for handheld wraps; use the smaller size if tortillas are to be stuffed, rolled, and baked, or layered and stacked. Choose between wheat and corn tortillas.

- Wheat tortillas are pliable, yet sturdy, so they're best for wraps, but they work well for anything.
- Corn tortillas often break when they're folded; use corn tortillas for baked recipes. Before filling, you'll need to soften them in sauce, such as tomato sauce or low-fat creamy soup.

Fillings. For quick tacos, wraps, and other filled tortillas that help you reach your calorie target, stock your kitchen with a variety of these ingredients.

- Canned beans. Refried beans are great in burritos; just add salsa. Look for the fat-free varieties. Drained kidney beans, chickpeas, black beans, and other canned beans make great filling "combos" with ground meat or veggies for Mexican dishes or international wraps with Greek, Asian, or Italian ingredients.
- Lean ground turkey or lean ground beef, boneless chicken breast, and lean stir-fry beef or pork for

your freezer. Cook these items first with a zesty seasoning, then use them for fajitas (stir-fried marinated chicken or meat and vegetables served in a warm flour tortilla), enchiladas (corn tortillas stuffed with beans, cheese, chicken, or meat and a sauce), burritos (flour tortillas that are folded, then rolled, to enclose the savory filling), or quesadillas (filled flour tortillas that are folded in half and then browned under a broiler). Or, for a tostada, layer tortillas with a filling of shredded lean meat or poultry.

- Canned crabmeat or tuna. Combined with rice, crabmeat or tuna is great for Asian-style wraps.
- Chopped frozen vegetables. Mix them into vegetarian tortilla wrap fillings or combine them with meat, chicken, or seafood filling.
- Cheese. For fewer calories, look for low-fat or fat-free varieties. Monterey Jack or jalapeño cheese is typical in many Mexican tortilla dishes. You can also find low-fat blends of shredded Mexican cheeses.

Sauces. Try tomato salsas with stir-fried meat, fruit salsas with stir-fried chicken, barbecue sauce with canned beans, picante sauce with chopped vegetables, and chutneys with cooked seafood.

Seasonings. Experiment with taco seasoning for Mexican fillings or barbecue wraps; ginger, soy sauce, and green onion for a California wrap; oregano, basil, and garlic for an Italian herb wrap.

Frozen tortilla dishes. Great for when time is even shorter. You'll find low-fat versions of burritos, enchiladas, and more in the freezer case. Check the label to compare the fat and calorie contents.

Weight-Friendly Substitutions

If stuffed soft tortillas are popular at your house, you've probably already thought of substituting fat-free cheese and sour cream for the full-fat versions. Here's what else you can do to enjoy your favorite combos while keeping calories and fat down.

- Use refried beans without fat, or mash your own, using any type of canned beans.
- Substitute salsa and yogurt cheese for guacamole and regular sour cream. (Make yogurt cheese by draining gelatin-free yogurt overnight until it is a thick consistency.)

Your Eating-Lean
Sample Meal Plan

To jump-start your shape-up efforts, follow this 1-week meal plan. Using food selections nutritionists rate as best, plus healthy recipes, you'll eat well and love it.

Each menu offers three tasty meals a day, plus snacks, for about 1,600 calories and less than 44 grams of fat (25 percent of total calories from fat).

These menus supply lots of flavor and variety (so you don't get bored) and fiber (so you feel satisfied and full and don't overeat). They also keep you fueled all day long, to maintain energy as you exercise regularly to lose weight and tone up. There's even plenty of room for extras, like sweets and treats.

With this menu, you can start paring off weight today while perking up classic family recipes and introducing exciting new foods into your menu. Break out of the rut of eating the same breakfast morning after morning, packing the same three lunch meals week in and week out, or cooking the same four family recipes over and over. Then use what you've learned to expand your weekly menu, using shopping, meal planning, and cooking strategies for eating lean.

Day 1

	Calories	Fat
Breakfast		
1 cup vanilla fortified soy milk mixed with	81	4.7
1 packet mocha instant breakfast powder	130	1
½ blueberry bagel	104	0.6
1 tablespoon whipped cream cheese	30	2.5
Snack		
1 tangerine	37	0.2
1 ounce pretzels	108	1
Lunch		
California-Style Turkey Burger (page 115)	289	2.6
on crusty roll with shredded lettuce and		
2 slices tomato		
1 cup broccoli coleslaw mix	25	0
2 tablespoons low-fat coleslaw dressing	22	0.4
Snack		
1 fresh pear	98	0.7
3 cups air-popped popcorn	90	0
Dinner		
Flounder Dijon (page 115)	184	3
½ cup boiled red potatoes tossed with	72	0.2
Dijon mustard and chopped chives		
½ cup peas with chopped mint	62	0.2
4 chocolate wafer cookies	104	3.6
1 cup orange sections	85	0.2
Snack		
1 cup 1% chocolate milk	158	2.5
Total	**1,679**	**23.4**
12.6 percent of calories from fat		

Day 2

	Calories	Fat
Breakfast		
1 sesame seed bagel, toasted	156	0.9
1 tablespoon apple butter	29	0
1 cup fat-free milk	86	0.4
Snack		
½ cup fresh blueberries	40	0.3
1 piece string cheese (1 ounce)	60	2.5
Lunch		
Pita Pizza (page 116)	247	5
1½ cups tossed spinach leaves and romaine lettuce	10	0.1
4 cherry tomatoes	14	0.2
2 tablespoons fat-free Italian dressing	20	0.3
Snack		
½ cup raisins	218	0.4
1 apple	81	0.5
Dinner		
1 serving *Baked Catfish with Dill Sauce* (page 117)	293	11
1 baked sweet potato, sprinkled with cinnamon	117	0.1
1 teaspoon soft margarine	34	3.8
½ cup steamed fresh green beans	22	0.2
1 whole wheat dinner roll	75	1.3
Snack		
8 ounces light cranberry juice cocktail	45	0
1 ounce pretzels	108	1
Total	1,615	28
15.6 percent of calories from fat		

Day 3

	Calories	Fat
Breakfast		
½ English muffin	134	1
1 tablespoon strawberry jam	56	0
½ grapefruit	41	0.1
1 cup fat-free milk	86	0.4
Snack		
3 cups air-popped popcorn	90	0
2 tablespoons grated Parmesan	46	3
Lunch		
Grilled Summer Salad (page 118)	132	1
¾ cup lemon sorbet	210	0
Snack		
6 graham crackers	178	4.2
1 cup fat-free milk	86	0.4
Dinner		
Jewel of the Nile Chicken Kabobs (page 119)	230	10
½ cup brown rice	108	0.9
⅛ wedge cantaloupe	36	0.3
Snack		
1 slice angel food cake	129	0.1
½ cup frozen strawberries, thawed	39	0.1
2 tablespoons nondairy topping	16	0.2
Total	1,617	21.7

12.1 percent of calories from fat

Day 4

	Calories	Fat
Breakfast		
½ grapefruit	41	0.1
1 slice whole wheat toast	70	1.1
1 tablespoon fruit spread	56	0
Snack		
¾ cup Concord grape juice	116	0.2
1 packet instant oatmeal	106	2.1
1 cup fat-free milk	86	0.4
Lunch		
Garden Vegetable Soup (page 120)	345	11
2 small whole-wheat pita	74	0.7
1 cup spinach salad	7	0.1
½ cup orange sections	42	0.2
Snack		
1 ounce reduced-fat Cheddar cheese	50	1.5
1 apple	81	0.5
Dinner		
Fettuccine with Pot-Lickin' Chicken Sauce (page 121)	429	6
½ cup steamed green beans	22	0.2
1 teaspoon slivered almonds	13	1.1
Snack		
1 cup tomato juice	41	0.1
4 whole-grain crackers	71	2.7
Total	1,650	28
15.3 percent of calories from fat		

Day 5

	Calories	Fat
Breakfast		
Easy Huevos Rancheros (page 121)	270	9
1 pear	98	0.7
Snack		
½ cup fat-free vanilla yogurt	60	0
½ cup low-fat granola	202	2.7
Lunch		
2 slices whole wheat bread	140	2.2
2 ounces reduced-fat mozzarella cheese	144	9
1 roasted bell pepper (packed in water)	6	0.1
fresh basil leaves	0	0
Snack		
¼ cup no-fat ranch dressing	86	0.6
½ cup cucumber slices	7	0
Dinner		
Grilled Garlicky Salmon (page 122)	268	14
1 cup brown rice	216	1.8
½ cup stewed tomatoes	36	0.2
1 cup steamed kale	36	0.5
Snack		
½ cup calcium-fortified orange juice	56	0.2
1 banana	108	0.6
Total	1,633	41.6

22.9 percent of calories from fat

Day 6

	Calories	Fat
Breakfast		
1 poached egg	74	5
Savory Hash Browns (page 123)	157	4
1 cup fat-free milk	86	0.4
Snack		
1 cup no-fat plain yogurt with	120	0
½ sliced banana	54	0.3
1 tablespoon chopped walnuts	47	4.4
Lunch		
1 cup cooked whole wheat pasta spirals	197	0.9
1 cup broccoli and yellow bell pepper	56	0.6
½ tomato, chopped	15	0.2
2 teaspoons olive oil and vinegar	42	4.5
Snack		
2 rye crispbread sheets	37	0.2
2 tablespoons light cream cheese	60	5
½ cup frozen strawberries, thawed	39	0.1
Dinner		
Shrimp Creole (page 124)	166	3
½ cup brown rice	108	0.9
1 cup curly endive	8	0
1 tablespoon crumbled bacon	36	3.1
1 tablespoon low-fat vinaigrette	16	1.5
1 wedge watermelon	92	1.2
Snack		
½ cup pear slices	48	0.3
½ cup fat-free cottage cheese	90	0
3 cups air-popped popcorn	90	0
Total	1,638	35.6
19.6 percent of calories from fat		

Day 7

	Calories	Fat
Breakfast		
Buttermilk Fruit Smoothie (page 125)	243	3
Snack		
1 serving instant chicken noodle soup	60	1
1 sesame bread stick	25	0.6
Lunch		
2 slices whole wheat bread	140	2.2
2 servings *Herbed Cheese Spread* (page 125)	64	4
½ cup alfalfa sprouts	5	0.1
Snack		
1 cup fat-free milk	86	0.4
3 whole graham crackers	117	4.2
Dinner		
Lentil-Sausage Stew (page 126)	568	15
1 cup romaine lettuce	8	0.1
1 tablespoon low-calorie vinaigrette	16	1.5
1 slice Italian bread	54	0.7
½ cup nonfat vanilla frozen yogurt	140	0
1 tablespoon chocolate syrup	52	0.2
Snack		
1 ounce caramel corn	122	3.6
Total	1,700	36.6

19.4 percent of calories from fat

California-Style Turkey Burgers

One of these tasty burgers has 13 grams of fat less than the same-size burger made of ground round. If you're serving fewer than 12, freeze the extra turkey mixture for future quick patties. Just form the patties, stack them (separated with pieces of wax paper), wrap well, and freeze.

3	pounds ground turkey breast
1	cup minced onion
1	cup celery
1	cup minced red bell pepper
¼	cup tomato paste
2	cloves garlic, minced
1	teaspoon ground black pepper
12	crusty rolls
	Shredded lettuce
	Tomato slices

In a large bowl, thoroughly mix the turkey, onion, celery, red pepper, tomato paste, garlic, and black pepper. Form into 12 patties. Grill, broil, or sauté until cooked through. Serve in the rolls with the lettuce and tomatoes.

Makes 12 servings

Per serving: 289 calories, 39 g protein, 26 g carbohydrates, 3 g fat, 95 mg cholesterol, 3 g fiber, 342 mg sodium

Flounder Dijon

Microwaving fish keeps it moist and gets dinner on the table in minutes.

4	large carrots, cut into matchsticks
2	tablespoons chopped parsley
1	teaspoon olive oil
⅛	teaspoon salt
⅛	teaspoon ground black pepper
4	flounder or cod fillets (¼ pound each)

> 2 teaspoons stone-ground Dijon mustard
> 1 teaspoon honey

In an 11" × 7" microwaveable dish, combine the carrots, parsley, oil, salt, and pepper. Cover with wax paper. Microwave on high power for 5 minutes, stirring once. Fold thin fillets to make each an even thickness. Place on top of the carrots in the corners of the dish, with the thickest parts toward the outside.

In a small bowl, combine the mustard and honey. Spread over the fish. Cover with wax paper. Microwave on high power for 2 minutes. Rotate the fillets, placing cooked parts toward the center, and cook for 1 to 3 minutes more, or just until the fish flakes easily. Let stand, covered, for 2 minutes.

Makes 4 servings
Per serving: 184 calories, 28 g protein, 9 g carbohydrates, 3 g fat, 77 mg cholesterol, 2 g fiber, 283 mg sodium

Pita Pizza
This is an update of the English muffin mini-pizzas from the 1950s.

> 4 small whole wheat or regular pitas
> ½ cup spaghetti sauce or tomato sauce
> 2 cups sliced vegetables (mushrooms, green peppers, tomatoes, onions)
> ½ cup shredded low-fat mozzarella cheese
> ½ teaspoon dried oregano
> 2 teaspoons extra-virgin olive oil

Preheat the oven to 450°F.
Split each pita into 2 thin rounds. Place, crust side down, on a large baking sheet. Bake for 10 minutes, or just until crisp.

Remove from the oven and top each round evenly with the sauce, vegetables, cheese, and oregano. Drizzle each with olive oil. Bake for 5 to 8 minutes, or just until the cheese melts.

Makes 4 servings

Per serving: 247 calories, 14 g protein, 43 g carbohydrates, 5 g fat, 0 mg cholesterol, 7 g fiber, 689 mg sodium

Baked Catfish with Dill Sauce

Farm-raised catfish is mild in flavor and low in fat. This simple recipe works well with other fish fillets.

¼	cup fat-free milk
2	catfish fillets (1½ pounds), cut into 4 pieces
1	cup fat-free plain yogurt
1	tablespoon dried dill
1	slice whole wheat bread
1	tablespoon melted butter or margarine
1	tablespoon Dijon mustard
¼	teaspoon salt

Preheat the oven to 325°F.

Pour the milk into a shallow baking dish. Then add the catfish.

In a cup, combine the yogurt and dill. Spread on top of the fish. Bake, uncovered, for 15 minutes.

Place the bread in a food processor or a blender and chop to make fine crumbs. Pour the crumbs into a small bowl and stir in the butter or margarine, mustard, and salt. Sprinkle over the fish. Bake for 10 minutes, or until the fish flakes easily and the crumbs brown.

Makes 4 servings

Per serving: 293 calories, 36 g protein, 10 g carbohydrates, 11 g fat, 107 mg cholesterol, 2 g fiber, 475 mg sodium

Grilled Summer Salad

This very low fat salad can be made ahead and served at room temperature. Remember it when you're grilling chicken or fish or even to dress up weeknight burgers.

Dressing

⅓   cup apricot preserves
⅓   cup balsamic vinegar
1   garlic clove, minced
1   teaspoon chopped fresh rosemary
¼   teaspoon salt

Salad

1   small eggplant, quartered lengthwise
1   large sweet onion, sliced ½" thick
1   large zucchini, sliced ½" thick
1   large red, yellow, or orange bell pepper, cut into strips
4   cups assorted salad greens (red leaf, Boston, arugula, watercress)

To make the dressing: In a small saucepan, combine the preserves, vinegar, garlic, rosemary, and salt. Heat to boiling over medium heat, stirring frequently. Remove from the heat.

To make the salad: Preheat the grill or broiler. Coat the grill rack or broiler pan with nonstick spray.

Grill the eggplant, onion, zucchini, and pepper over medium-high heat or broil 4" from the heat for 8 to 10 minutes, or until tender. Turn the vegetables occasionally and brush with the dressing. Serve over the greens. Pour any remaining dressing over the vegetables.

Makes 4 servings

Per serving: 132 calories, 6 g protein, 29 g carbohydrates, 1 g fat, 0 mg cholesterol, 5 g fiber, 500 mg sodium

Jewel of the Nile Chicken Kabobs

These kabobs are always a hit. The colorful vegetables are like jewels on a skewer, and the marinade gives them a Middle Eastern flavor. They make great party fare, too.

¼	cup chopped parsley
¼	cup fat-free plain yogurt
¼	cup lemon juice
2	tablespoons olive oil
1	tablespoon chopped fresh cilantro
1	tablespoon paprika
1	tablespoon curry powder
2	teaspoons ground cumin
2	small garlic cloves, minced
½	teaspoon salt
½	teaspoon ground black pepper
1	pound boneless, skinless chicken breasts, cubed
1	small yellow or orange bell pepper, cut into 1" pieces
1	yellow summer squash, sliced ¼" thick
8	cherry tomatoes
1	onion, cut into ½" wedges

In a large bowl, combine the parsley, yogurt, lemon juice, oil, cilantro, paprika, curry powder, cumin, garlic, salt, and black pepper. Add the chicken and toss to coat. Cover and refrigerate for at least 20 minutes or up to 2 hours.

Heat a large saucepan of lightly salted water to boiling. Drop in the bell pepper and cook for 2 minutes. Remove with a slotted spoon and drain. Drop in the squash and cook for 1 minute. Remove with a slotted spoon and drain. Thread a cherry tomato onto each of 4 skewers, then alternately thread the marinated chicken, bell pepper, squash, and onion, ending with a cherry tomato.

Coat a grill rack or broiler pan with nonstick spray. Preheat the grill or broiler. Grill kabobs 4" to 6" from the heat for 3 to 4 minutes per side, or until the chicken is no longer pink when tested with a sharp knife.

Makes 4 servings
Per serving: 230 calories, 21 g protein, 16 g carbohydrates, 10 g fat, 46 mg cholesterol, 4 g fiber, 344 mg sodium

Garden Vegetable Soup

This veggie soup is chock-full of goodies, and the servings are generous. The soy sauce gives it a shot of big flavor. Beets add a pleasant rosy color.

2	tablespoons oil
1	large onion, chopped
3	cans (14½ ounces each) reduced-sodium chicken broth
2	carrots, sliced
2	celery ribs, finely chopped
2	potatoes, cut into 1" cubes
2	beets, peeled and cut into 1" cubes
1	cup green beans cut into 1" pieces
¼	head green cabbage, shredded
2	garlic cloves, minced
1	bay leaf
1	tablespoon soy sauce
1	cup fresh or frozen green peas

Warm the oil in a large soup pot over medium heat. Add the onion and cook for 5 minutes, or until tender. Add the broth, carrots, celery, potatoes, beets, beans, cabbage, garlic, bay leaf, and soy sauce. Heat to boiling. Reduce the heat to low and simmer for 15 minutes. Stir in the peas and cook for 10 minutes. Remove and discard the bay leaf before serving.

Makes 4 servings
Per serving: 345 calories, 11 g protein, 55 g carbohydrates, 11 g fat, 0 mg cholesterol, 12 g fiber, 417 mg sodium

Fettuccine with Pot-Lickin' Chicken Sauce

When you want a healthy alternative to regular meat sauce, use skinless chicken pieces instead of fatty ground beef.

1	tablespoon olive oil
1	pound boneless, skinless chicken breast, cubed
1	green bell pepper, chopped
1	can (28 ounces) tomatoes packed in puree, or crushed tomatoes
1	small onion, quartered
4	garlic cloves
2	teaspoons sugar
2	teaspoons dried basil
½	teaspoon ground black pepper
1	can (4 ounces) pitted, sliced black olives, drained (optional)
8	ounces dried fettuccine

Warm the oil in large saucepan over medium-high heat. Add the chicken and bell pepper. Cook for 5 minutes.

In a blender, combine the tomatoes (with juice), onion, garlic, sugar, basil, and black pepper. Blend until smooth. Add to the chicken. Reduce the heat to medium-low and simmer for 25 minutes, or until slightly thickened. Stir in the olives, if using.

Cook the fettuccine according to the package directions. Drain and serve topped with the chicken sauce.

Makes 4 servings

Per serving: 429 calories, 28 g protein, 64 g carbohydrates, 6 g fat, 46 mg cholesterol, 6 g fiber, 534 mg sodium

Easy Huevos Rancheros

Treat yourself with this simplified version of a traditional egg dish. It's especially quick, and everything (except for poaching the eggs) is done right on the baking sheet that goes under the broiler.

4 large eggs
4 corn tortillas (6" diameter)
1 cup canned refried beans
½ cup salsa
¼ cup shredded reduced-fat Cheddar cheese

Preheat the broiler. Lightly coat a baking sheet with nonstick spray.

In a medium skillet or saucepan, heat 1½" water to boiling. Reduce the heat to low. Gently break the eggs into the simmering water. Cook for 3 to 5 minutes, or until the whites are set.

Place the tortillas on the prepared baking sheet and heat under the broiler for 1 minute, or until slightly crisp but not brown. Flip the tortillas and spread the untoasted sides with the refried beans. Return to the broiler and cook for 1 minute, or just until heated through. Top each tortilla with a poached egg, 2 tablespoons of salsa, and 1 tablespoon of cheese. Return to the broiler and cook for 30 seconds, or just until the cheese melts.

Makes 4 servings
Per serving: 270 calories, 16 g protein, 31 g carbohydrates, 9 g fat, 223 mg cholesterol, 3 g fiber, 677 mg sodium

Grilled Garlicky Salmon
Basil vinaigrette gives this summery salmon a great aroma. Grilling over hot coals intensifies the taste. You can also broil it 3" to 4" from the heat.

2 tablespoons red wine vinegar
2 tablespoons finely chopped fresh basil
1 tablespoon olive oil
2 garlic cloves, minced
4 salmon steaks or fillets (6 ounces each)

In a large baking dish, combine the vinegar, basil, oil, and garlic. Add the salmon and turn to coat. Cover and refrigerate for at least 15 minutes or up to 2 hours.

Coat a grill rack with nonstick spray. Preheat the grill.

Grill the salmon for 10 minutes per inch of thickness, turning halfway through the cooking time.

Makes 4 servings
Per serving: 268 calories, 33 g protein, 1 g carbohydrates, 14 g fat, 91 mg cholesterol, 0 g fiber, 73 mg sodium

Savory Hash Browns
The secret to crispy hash browns is to cook the potatoes without peeling them. The skins give a rustic flavor and add fiber, too.

1	tablespoon oil
2	baking potatoes, coarsely shredded
1	small onion, coarsely shredded
1	garlic clove, minced
¾	teaspoon salt
¼	teaspoon ground black pepper

Warm the oil in a large nonstick skillet over medium heat.

In a large bowl, combine the potatoes, onion, garlic, salt, and pepper. Spread evenly in the skillet. Top with a 9" or 10" plate or cake pan weighted down with something heavy, such as cans of soup. Cook for 4 minutes, or until browned. Turn potatoes over and cook for 4 minutes, or until browned.

Makes 4 servings
Per serving: 157 calories, 3 g protein, 29 g carbohydrates, 4 g fat, 0 mg cholesterol, 1 g fiber, 409 mg sodium

Shrimp Creole

Here's a lower-fat way to enjoy this classic dish. Serve over hot cooked rice.

2	bacon strips
1	onion, chopped
½	green bell pepper, chopped
1	celery rib, chopped
1	garlic clove, minced
1	can (16 ounces) chopped tomatoes
1	bay leaf
½	teaspoon salt
¼	teaspoon ground black pepper
¼	teaspoon Worcestershire sauce
¼	teaspoon hot-pepper sauce
1	pound medium shrimp, peeled and deveined

Cook the bacon in a large skillet over medium heat until crisp. Remove bacon to paper towels. Crumble when cool. Remove and discard all but 1 tablespoon of the drippings from the skillet.

Add the onion, bell pepper, and celery. Cook over medium heat for 5 minutes, or until tender. Stir in the garlic and cook for 1 minute. Add the tomatoes (with juice), bay leaf, salt, black pepper, Worcestershire sauce, and hot-pepper sauce. Heat to boiling. Reduce the heat to low and simmer for 20 minutes. Add the shrimp and bacon. Cook for 10 minutes, or until the shrimp are opaque. Remove and discard the bay leaf before serving.

Makes 4 servings

Per serving: 166 calories, 22 g protein, 12 g carbohydrates, 3 g fat, 178 mg cholesterol, 3 g fiber, 820 mg sodium

Buttermilk Fruit Smoothie

The refreshing creaminess of this shake comes from the buttermilk. But it's also good made with fat-free milk or low-fat soy milk. Use your favorite frozen fruit or a combination of fruits.

    2   cups low-fat buttermilk
    1   ripe banana, cut into chunks
    1   cup frozen unsweetened strawberries or peaches
    2   tablespoons honey
    1   cup ice cubes

In a blender combine the buttermilk, banana, strawberries or peaches, honey, and ice. Blend until frothy.

Makes 2 servings
Per serving: 243 calories, 9 g protein, 49 g carbohydrates, 3 g fat, 9 mg cholesterol, 3 g fiber, 264 mg sodium

Herbed Cheese Spread

There's no need to give up cheese when you have this easy spread on hand. Serve with soda crackers or Belgian endive.

    1   cup fat-free sour cream
    1   cup shredded reduced-fat Cheddar cheese
    1   scallion, minced
    2   tablespoons chopped parsley
    ½   teaspoon dried thyme
    ½   teaspoon dried rosemary, crushed
    ½   teaspoon ground black pepper

In a medium bowl, combine the sour cream, cheese, scallion, parsley, thyme, rosemary, and pepper. Cover and refrigerate up to 4 days.

Makes 2 cups
Per 2 tablespoons: 32 calories, 3 g protein, 2 g carbohydrates, 2 g fat, 5 mg cholesterol, 0 g fiber, 45 mg sodium

Lentil-Sausage Stew

Even sausage can fit into a slimming eating plan!

1	tablespoon olive oil
1	onion, chopped
1	green bell pepper, chopped
1	pound turkey sausage, crumbled, or reduced-fat kielbasa, thinly sliced
3	garlic cloves, minced
2	cups dry lentils
2	cups fat-free reduced-sodium chicken broth
1	can (14 ounces) low-sodium tomatoes
1	teaspoon fennel seeds
½	teaspoon dried Italian seasoning
½	teaspoon dried thyme
½	teaspoon ground black pepper

Warm the oil in a large nonstick skillet over medium heat. Add the onion and bell pepper. Cook for 10 minutes. Stir in the sausage or kielbasa and garlic. Cook for 10 minutes, stirring occasionally. Stir in the lentils, broth, tomatoes (with juice), fennel seeds, Italian seasoning, thyme, and black pepper. Heat to boiling. Reduce the heat to low, cover, and simmer for 40 minutes, or until the lentils are tender.

Makes 4 servings

Per serving: 568 calories, 48 g protein, 69 g carbohydrates, 15 g fat, 71 mg cholesterol, 2 g fiber, 1,067 mg sodium

Low-Fat Cooking
Techniques

The beauty of healthy cooking is that it's both simple and fast. It doesn't require a lot of exotic ingredients. It often uses brief cooking times to enhance flavors and preserve vitamins and minerals. And you don't have to load your kitchen cabinets with a lot of expensive cookware.

At its most basic, healthy cooking doesn't need much more than a steamer basket, a wok, maybe a grill, a few sauté pans, and a couple of pots for boiling water. Add a slow cooker and a microwave and there's nothing you won't be able to do.

Three of the most common techniques—stir-frying, sautéing, and poaching—are among the fastest. Grilling takes a little more time, but only because you have to wait for the grill to heat up. Once your meats and vegetables are prepared and the grill is hot, the actual cooking time is usually less than 10 minutes.

In the following pages, we take a look at these and a few other healthy-cooking techniques.

Stir-Frying

Stir-frying is among the simplest of all kitchen techniques. It doesn't require anything more than a wok or high-sided skillet, and it's fast. Once you've cut up the ingredients, most meals are done in 5 minutes or less.

There's a good reason why healthy cooks do a lot of stir-frying. This technique essentially "flash-cooks" food, so you don't need to add much cooking oil, says Deann Bayless, chef and owner of the Frontera Grill in Chicago. Fresh foods retain their natural colors, textures, and freshness. Meats are by no means excluded from stir-fries, but most recipes call for an abundance of vegetables, fresh as well as frozen. And because it's all cooked in one pan, there's very little cleanup time.

As with all fast-cooking methods, stir-frying isn't recommended for tough foods or foods in big pieces. Yet even tough foods can be made tender enough for stir-frying just by cutting them thin and cooking them quickly.

Begin with a wok. Although deep-sided skillets are adequate for stir-fries, woks are better because the higher sides speed cooking time and allow more room for foods to cook, says Jackie Newgent, R.D., a nutrition and culinary consultant in New York City and spokesperson for the American Dietetic Association. The best woks cook on the stove top; electric models don't get hot enough for efficient stir-frying. Many cooks prefer flat-bottomed woks, which sit solidly on electric and gas heating elements. Round-bottomed woks are fine, but you'll need to use a metal ring (which may or may not be included when you buy the wok) to give them stability.

Prepare ingredients ahead of time. Stir-fry cooking is extremely fast, so you won't have time to prepare ingredients as you work.

Stir early and often. Stirring, as the name *stir-fry* suggests, is central to this cooking technique. Allowing food to stay in one place will cause it to absorb fluids and lose its fresh, crisp texture. While food is cooking in one place, the wok is getting hotter somewhere else. Frequent stirring moves food from hot spot to hot spot so that it cooks more quickly.

Marinate the meat. Since you'll be using lean meats when making stir-fries, it helps to slice them thinly and marinate them for 10 to 15 minutes before you start cooking. To create a simple marinade, combine ¼ cup soy sauce, 2 tablespoons vinegar (such as red wine, white wine, or rice), 1 tablespoon honey, and a chopped clove of garlic.

Keep tofu firm. Tofu is a popular ingredient in stir-fries because it adds protein and other nutrients to meatless meals, and it soaks up the flavors of whatever it's cooked with. It's best to use the firm style of tofu, which holds its shape better.

Go for crisp textures. Stir-fry cooking is designed to sear the outer surfaces of food and heat the pieces through. It's not designed for long, slow cooking. So keep an eye on vegetables and other ingredients. "Don't overcook them," says Newgent. "You want a bit of crispness."

Sautéing

The word *sautéed* is often followed by the phrase "with butter." While traditional sautés do in fact use butter, sometimes in artery-clogging amounts, fat isn't an integral part of this very healthy cooking process. In some ways sautéing is similar to stir-frying, in that fairly small pieces of food are cooked quickly.

Sautéing is very fast. Food is cooked at high temperatures, although generally not quite so hot as those used in stir-fries.

Ingredients are often sautéed as part of a recipe. For example, onions, garlic, and mushrooms are typically sautéed, then added to other ingredients that will undergo further cooking. Boneless chicken breast and pork tenderloin, on the other hand, may be sautéed for a simple, easy-to-prepare meal.

Get a heavy pan. Sautéing requires a bit of stirring, and pans that are too light will skate all over the stove and cause scorching or uneven cooking. The best sauté pans are tin-lined copper skillets. They're heavy and they conduct heat quickly and evenly. They're very expensive, however, which is why many cooks choose cast-iron skillets, which also hold and conduct heat well.

Reduce fat by preparing the pan. Since healthy sautés use very little fat, prepare the surface of cast-iron pans before cooking to make sure that food doesn't stick. It takes only a second. Pour a teaspoon of salt into the cool pan, scour it around with a paper towel, then pour it out. Follow this with a light film of oil, then wipe the pan well with a paper towel. The almost invisible sheen of oil will help food cook evenly without sticking.

Invest in nonstick pans. When you're really serious about reducing the amount of oil you cook with, buy a set of nonstick pots and pans. Even if you don't use any oil, the food glides across the surface rather than sticking.

Older generations of nonstick pans scratched easily, and the marred surfaces allowed foods to stick. The newer pans are much more rugged. Some are guaranteed to maintain their special finish for decades, and they're designed to withstand high heats as well as metal implements. These pans are expensive, but they're worth it because there's a good chance you'll never have to replace them.

Leave plenty of empty space. For sautés to cook quickly and evenly, place pieces of meat or poultry in a single layer with lots of space in between.

Leave it alone. The point of sautéing is to let food cook to a perfect golden brown. Let it cook, undisturbed, for a few minutes in one place. Then move it to another part of the pan for further cooking. This has the added advantage of preventing sticking.

Poaching

The gentlest of cooking methods, poaching occurs when food is submerged in hot liquid and carefully simmered until it's done. Often foods are poached as a prelude to further preparation. Chicken breasts may be poached before being sliced and added to cold chicken salad. Poaching can also be the main cooking method for delicate, tender foods such as fish.

Use a deep enough pan. You can poach in any skillet or pot as long as it's deep enough to allow the cooking liquid to completely cover the food. Don't use a cast-iron skillet, however, because iron absorbs flavors and may impart an "off" taste to mild foods.

Flavor the liquid. Since poached foods are naturally mild, it's important to add flavors to the cooking liquid itself. The easiest way to season poaching liquid is to combine reduced-sodium chicken broth or wine with lemon juice and rosemary or other herbs. This works very well for chicken or fish.

Keep the water action gentle. Rigorous boiling will cause tender foods to toughen or fall apart. The liquid should be at a very gentle simmer.

Wrap delicate foods in cheesecloth. It can be tricky to get a whole fish into and out of the poaching liquid without having it fall apart. Wrapping it in cheesecloth before submerging it in the liquid will help it hold its shape without interfering with the poaching.

Start fish cold and chicken hot. When poaching a whole fish, it's best to start it in cold liquid so the skin won't split. For chicken or fish fillets, it's fine to add them to liquid that's already simmering.

Steaming

Moist heat cooks food gently with no added fat. In addition, it allows foods to retain most of their original character. Vegetables taste fresh-picked and keep their shape, texture, and brilliant colors. Fish and seafood maintain their delicate flavors. And poultry, even when you take off the skin, cooks up plump, juicy, and moist.

Steaming cooks food quickly because temperatures rise above 212°F, the boiling point of water. This helps tenderize food while locking in moisture and nutrients. And because cooking takes place *over* water rather than in it, vitamins are retained that might otherwise wash away.

Use any kind of steamer. All steamers work in roughly the same way. If you do a lot of steaming, you may want to invest in a bamboo or stainless steel multitiered steamer. For most foods, however, inexpensive collapsible metal steamer baskets, which drop into any pan deep enough to hold them, work just as well.

Start your timing late. Once food is added to a steamer, the temperature of the water drops, and it will need a minute or two to return to a boil. Start your timing from the moment the water begins boiling again.

Don't let curiosity slow you down. Trapped steam cooks the food. Every time you open the lid, steam escapes and substantially slows the cooking time.

Add additional flavors. The moist environment inside a steamer dilutes herbs and spices, so you may want to add more than usual. Rather than spice the food itself, you can add herbs or spices to the water to impart subtle flavors.

Protect yourself. Always open the steamer cover away from yourself to prevent burns.

Grilling

Grilling is the opposite of steaming. It uses dry heat, not moist. It imparts a lot of its own flavors rather than merely bringing out a food's natural flavors. And for the most part, it works best with robust foods. For healthy cooks who don't have a lot of time, it has the advantage of cooking most foods very quickly without much additional fat.

Begin with a marinade. Because grilling is a dry process, most meats benefit from a marinade or a basting liquid. The difference between the two is that foods soak in marinades, while you brush on bastes during cooking. Ideally, poultry and meat should marinate in the refrigerator for a few hours before cooking.

"Marinades do not need fat," Newgent adds. She recommends mixing herbs and spices in an acidic liquid—such as vinegar, citrus juice, or even wine—which will tenderize the meat.

Start with a hot grill. Putting meat, fish, or poultry on a cold grill makes the food more likely to stick. You can prevent this by cleaning the grill thoroughly when it's cool, then adding the food once the grill is hot.

Grill chicken with the skin on. Grilling tends to dry foods out. Cooking chicken in the skin essentially makes it self-basting. The meat itself absorbs little of the fat, however, so you'll still have a healthy meal once you remove the skin after cooking.

Consider precooking poultry. Unless you're grilling thin strips, chicken can take a while to grill, so it's helpful to precook it by poaching, baking, or microwaving immediately before putting it on the grill.

Add some smoke. Hardwood chips, dried herbs, or citrus rinds can be added to the coals or lava rocks to impart a smoky flavor that complements most grilled foods. When using smoke chips, close the grill lid to get the most intense flavors.

Combine grilling and steaming. Wrapping ears of corn, fish, or poultry in foil and adding seasoning and a little water makes it possible to get the fast-cooking benefits of steaming along with the flavors from the grill.

PART THREE

Body-Shaping Workouts

Trimming Your Tummy

Donna Michaels never used to worry about her abdomen.

The former bodybuilder from Miami expects to look in the mirror and see well-defined muscles etched into her midsection. But as she approaches her fifties, Michaels notices a belly that she never thought she would have. She had always carried her weight on her hips and thighs—a classic pear shape. Until now.

"Now that I'm older, my abdomen is betraying me," she states.

As a certified personal trainer, fitness director, and author of *Underneath It All: Either You Live It or You Diet*, Michaels knows what she needs to do: With every year, she'll have to work smarter (not harder) to keep her tummy flat. That's because she is nearing menopause, one of the most common belly bloaters.

"It's not impossible to control abdominal fat at my age. But it is a little more difficult," says Michaels. "I can't let abdominal exercise slide."

The Two Enemies of a Tight Tummy

Menopause can have a dramatic effect on the shape of a woman's body. Women who have fought off hip fat for most of their lives hit menopause and find a new foe, tummy fat.

Researchers are not entirely sure why. But the drop in the female sex hormones that coincides with menopause may have something to do with the change in fat patterning, says Claude Bouchard, Ph.D., professor of exercise physiology at Laval University in Ste. Foy, Quebec.

Menopause isn't the only life event that bulges bellies. Pregnancy also creates problems. As the baby grows inside the womb, the surrounding abdominal muscles stretch. And stretch.

Muscles consist of proteins that are woven together in the shape of a ladder. When the muscle is overstretched, the proteins that form the sides of the ladder move away from the proteins that form the steps, says Diane Habash, Ph.D., nutrition research manager in the General Clinic Research Center at Ohio State University in Columbus.

As the proteins separate, they lose not only their strength but also their elasticity. The problem grows if you have another baby, or if you have a cesarean section, which also weakens abdominal muscles by slicing them apart. The result of all that abdominal stress is that your muscles have trouble performing even the most basic duty: holding your internal organs in place.

That's news that's hard to stomach. "But abdominal exercises can get your abdomen as strong as before," says Dr. Habash.

The Three Areas You Can't Neglect

When you exercise your abdominal muscles, you make them tighter. The tighter they are, the more they hold in your stomach and other internal organs so that they don't protrude, explains Rudolph Leibel, M.D., associate professor at the laboratory of human behavior and metabolism at Rockefeller University in New York City.

But all the abdominal exercises in the world won't help you reduce a potbelly unless you combine them with fat-burning aerobic exercise and a calorie-zapping total-body strength-training program, according to Michael Pollock, Ph.D., professor of medicine and exercise science at the University of Florida in Gainesville. That's because a big middle is caused not only by sagging organs but also by the fat that surrounds them. Abdominal work will shape up your midsection as you're whittling away your fat.

And when it comes to the abdominal work, *quality* counts more than *quantity*. To get a flat tummy, experts say you need to work three different areas: the upper rectus abdominis, the lower abdominals, and the obliques.

Plenty of women work the upper rectus abdominis, the portion of this muscle that runs from the belly button to the rib cage, says Mia Finnegan, a Fitness America Pageant National Champion and Miss Olympia Fitness, who with her husband operates a training service called Tru Fitness in Pasadena, California. But fewer women work the obliques, the muscles that travel diagonally along the sides of the torso. And even fewer women work the lower abdominal muscle, which lies below the belly button. Yet the lower abdominal area is where most women notice a bulge, she notes.

How do you work those areas? Traditional crunches do little to work your obliques or the lower abdomen, which is why you may have failed at flattening your tummy even if you did as many as 200 situps a day. To work your obliques, you need to modify a traditional crunch by adding a twist, or try other twisting movements. To work your lower abdominals, you can tilt your pelvis while raising and lowering your legs, according to Finnegan.

If you have back problems, consult your doctor before doing these exercises. If you have back pain or discomfort while doing these, stop immediately and consult your doctor, advises Dr. Pollock.

Exercises: A 30-Day Beginner Program

Here's a 4-week program to get those muscles in shape. Do each exercise three times per week for the recommended number of repetitions. As you get fitter, move from the beginner's number of reps to the intermediate level. Then progress to the 30-day intermediate program below.

Week 1

Curl-Ups 1 (page 155). *Beginner:* 1 set of 3 to 10 reps, 3 days per week. *Intermediate:* 2 sets of 10 reps, 3 days per week.

Pelvic Tilts (page 160). *Beginner:* 1 set of 3 to 10 reps, 3 days per week. *Intermediate:* 2 sets of 10 reps, 3 days per week.

Side Bends (page 164). *Beginner:* 1 set of 3 to 10 reps on each side, 3 days per week. *Intermediate:* 2 sets of 10 reps on each side, 3 days per week.

Week 2

Pelvic Tilts (page 160). *Beginner:* 1 set of 3 to 10 reps, 3 days per week. *Intermediate:* 2 sets of 10 reps, 3 days per week.

Side Bends (page 164). *Beginner:* 1 set of 3 to 10 reps on each side, 3 days per week. *Intermediate:* 2 sets of 10 reps on each side, 3 days per week.

Curl-Ups 1 (page 155). *Beginner:* 1 set of 3 to 10 reps, 3 days per week. *Intermediate:* 2 sets of 10 reps, 3 days per week.

Week 3

Diagonal Curl-Ups 1 (page 162). *Beginner:* 1 set of 3 to 10 reps on each side, 3 days per week. *Intermediate:* 2 sets of 10 reps on each side, 3 days per week.

Curl-Ups 1 (page 155). *Beginner:* 1 set of 3 to 10 reps, 3 days per week. *Intermediate:* 2 sets of 10 reps, 3 days per week.

Pelvic Tilts (page 160). *Beginner:* 1 set of 3 to 10 reps, 3 days per week. *Intermediate:* 2 sets of 10 reps, 3 days per week.

Week 4

Knee-Up Crunches (page 157). *Beginner:* 1 set of 3 to 10 reps, 3 days per week. *Intermediate:* 2 sets of 10 reps, 3 days per week.

Diagonal Curl-Ups 1 (page 162). *Beginner:* 1 set of 3 to 10 reps on each side, 3 days per week. *Intermediate:* 2 sets of 10 reps on each side, 3 days per week.

Modified Knee Raises (page 159). *Beginner:* 1 set of 3 to 10 reps, 3 days per week. *Intermediate:* 2 sets of 10 reps, 3 days per week.

Exercises: A 30-Day Intermediate Program

As you gain strength, switch to this program.

Week 1

Curl-Ups 2 (page 156). *Beginner:* 1 set of 3 to 10 reps, 3 days per week. *Intermediate:* 2 sets of 10 reps, 3 days per week.

Diagonal Curl-Ups 2 (page 163). *Beginner:* 1 set of 3 to 10 reps on each side, 3 days per week. *Intermediate:* 2 sets of 10 reps on each side, 3 days per week.

Reverse Curls (page 161). *Beginner:* 1 set of 3 to 10 reps, 3 days per week. *Intermediate:* 2 sets of 10 reps, 3 days per week.

Week 2

Reverse Curls (page 161). *Beginner:* 1 set of 3 to 10 reps, 3 days per week. *Intermediate:* 2 sets of 10 reps, 3 days per week.

Curl-Ups 2 (page 156). *Beginner:* 1 set of 3 to 10 reps, 3 days per week. *Intermediate:* 2 sets of 10 reps, 3 days per week.

Diagonal Curl-Ups 2 (page 163). *Beginner:* 1 set of 3 to 10 reps on each side, 3 days per week. *Intermediate:* 2 sets of 10 reps on each side, 3 days per week.

Week 3

Reverse Curls (page 161). *Beginner:* 1 set of 3 to 10 reps, 3 days per week. *Intermediate:* 2 sets of 10 reps, 3 days per week.

Diagonal Curl-Ups 2 (page 163). *Beginner:* 1 set of 3 to 10 reps on each side, 3 days per week. *Intermediate:* 2 sets of 10 reps on each side, 3 days per week.

Curl-Ups 2 (page 156). *Beginner:* 1 set of 3 to 10 reps, 3 days per week. *Intermediate:* 2 sets of 10 reps, 3 days per week.

Week 4

Curl-Ups 2 (page 156). *Beginner:* 1 set of 3 to 10 reps, 3 days per week. *Intermediate:* 2 sets of 10 reps, 3 days per week.

Hip Raises (page 158). *Beginner:* 1 set of 3 to 10 reps, 3 days per week. *Intermediate:* 2 sets of 10 reps, 3 days per week.

Side Jackknives (page 165). *Beginner:* 1 set of 3 to 10 reps on each side, 3 days per week. *Intermediate:* 2 sets of 10 reps on each side, 3 days per week.

Tightening Your Butt
and Thighs

By many women's standards, Carrie Givens wasn't what you would call overweight. Before she had children, she weighed a mere 100 pounds. Even at the age of 43, the petite mother of three weighed just 117 pounds. Problem was, the extra pounds seemed to have accumulated on her hips and thighs.

"I was definitely pear-shaped," says Carrie, an art teacher in Alliance, Ohio, whose three daughters are now 13, 15, and 19. "I felt frumpy."

Carrie blamed her heavy hips and thighs on heredity, having children, and age. She tried to lose weight. She also tried running and swimming, but she wasn't very consistent. Carrie just couldn't seem to trim her hips and thighs—until she started to work out with weights.

"My sister owns a fitness center, and she encouraged me to try weight training," says Carrie. "I started doing leg raises, curls, extensions, and lunges 3 days a week. I lost inches on my hips and thighs, but especially my thighs."

In addition, Carrie spends time on a step machine, for 5 to 15 minutes a session, or she does a 40-minute aerobic class to warm up. And she's more consistent about aerobic exercise. "I run, bike, and take aerobics classes. But the weight training has made the most significant difference in my thighs," she says.

Carrie also follows a more structured low-fat diet, which includes lots of fruits, vegetables, cereal, and soy milk. For protein, she eats fish and tofu and a little red meat.

After 6 months of working out with weights, she weighs 110 pounds. But to Carrie, the important thing is that she lost fat and gained muscle.

Thinner, Shapelier Hips and Thighs

Carrie's quest for thinner hips and thighs is shared by many women.

"Most women, even if they're not overly pear-shaped, will gain weight in their hips and thighs before they gain it anywhere else," points out Marjorie Albohm, an exercise physiologist, certified athletic trainer, and director of sports medicine at Kendrick Memorial Hospital in Mooresville, Indiana.

Heavier hips, thighs, and buttocks are a factor more of gender than of age. "Whether they're 20 or 40, women still have 10 to 15 percent more body fat than men, even if they work out," says Albohm. As for the myth that sitting at a desk is responsible for wider hips and a broader backside—the so-called secretary spread—that's just not true, she says.

"Sitting itself doesn't necessarily determine where fat is deposited," says Albohm. "Our sedentary lifestyle in general does that. Your muscles would be far more toned if you were active—working on a farm, climbing up and down ladders, and so forth. Those are the exercises that tone the muscles in your hips and thighs."

Done correctly, cutting dietary fat and calories can help you lose weight overall, and that can certainly help "shrink" your hips, thighs, and buttocks to some degree. So can aerobic exercise, which burns excess body fat and calories as you work your heart and lungs, like walking, jogging, biking, or taking aerobics classes. Purposeful exercise can make up for the kind of sedentary lifestyle that packs pounds on overall, including on the hips and thighs. But to see a real difference in your lower body, says Albohm, you have to do what Carrie did—add resistance training to the mix.

Muscles Meant to Be Worked

The muscles that form the hips, thighs, and buttocks include:

- The gluteal muscles (small, medium, and large muscles that form the buttocks)
- The quadriceps (the muscles on the front of the thighs)
- The hamstrings (the muscles on the back of the thighs)
- The abductors (the outer thighs)
- The adductors (the inner thighs)

In some women, the thigh muscles are long and lean; in others, they're shorter and broader. "So again, genetics is a primary factor in the size and shape of your thighs," says Albohm. But so is use (or lack thereof).

The gluteals, quadriceps, and hamstrings are the "worker" muscles—the ones you'd use if you led a life of running, jumping, climbing, and lifting heavy objects. The adductors, in particular, suffer from neglect.

To tone and trim your hips, thighs, and buttocks, "you need a total-body workout with special emphasis on the muscle groups that you want to tone," says Albohm. "Your goal is to change the circumference of this area." Combined with some kind of consistent aerobic exercise—and eating habits that subtract pounds—the workout programs that follow can help you reach your goal, she says. If you're just starting to exercise, start with the beginner exercises. If you are able to complete a designated program with relative ease for three consecutive workout sessions, then it's time to proceed to the next level.

You can expect to see some change in as little as 30 days, says Albohm.

Working Smart

As with any exercise, there's a right and a wrong way to go about working your hips, thighs, and buttocks.

Easy does it—at first. Start with the beginner program until you get used to the movements, says Albohm. If you decide to add ankle weights to work your inner and outer thigh muscles, start with light weights and only a few reps. Don't exceed 5 pounds—if you do so, you completely change the leverage on your joints.

Do the exercise correctly, to avoid injury. If you arch your back while you're doing the hip extension, for example, you could strain your back. And don't cheat—complete the full range of motion.

Make yourself comfortable. For some of the exercises that are done on the floor, you'll probably want to use an exercise mat. If you don't have a mat, a carpeted floor or folded large towel may work just as well. But if you experience pain or discomfort when performing an exercise, stop and substitute another version, advises Albohm. If pain persists, see your physician.

Keep your movements tight and controlled. Don't swing your way through the exercise or let your muscles go slack.

Work your whole body. "Despite what you may have heard, if aerobic exercise is strenuous enough—if you walk like you really mean it, for example—it can tone your muscles to some degree," says Albohm. "I do aerobics primarily for the cardiovascular effects, for example. But 20 to 30 percent of my effort carries over to strengthen and tone my muscles."

Step right up. Step aerobics is better for the hips, thighs, and buttocks than regular aerobics because it involves the quads, adductors, abductors, and gluteals, says Albohm. Stairclimbing machines work the quads, hamstrings, and gluteals, without overstressing the hips—you work up and down in a straight line.

If you use a stairclimber, program the machine to vary the resistance and height to give your muscles a thorough workout, recommends Albohm. (The same advice applies if you use an elliptical trainer or a recumbent bike.)

Measure your progress. It's a good idea to measure your hips, thighs, and buttocks every month, not every week, says Albohm. "Just be sure to measure at the same spot, in the same way, every time." And don't worry that your hips, thighs, and buttocks will get bigger when you follow this program. These exercises don't do that.

Be consistent. To get the fastest results in the shortest period of time, do the exercises exactly as shown.

Exercises: A 30-Day Beginner Program

Here's a 4-week program to get those muscles in shape. Do each exercise three times per week for the recommended number of repetitions. As you get fitter, move from the beginner's number of reps to the intermediate level. Then progress to the 30-day intermediate program below.

Week 1

Leg Extensions (page 166). *Beginner:* 3 to 10 reps with each leg, 3 days per week. *Intermediate:* 2 sets of 10 reps with each leg, 3 days per week.

Leg Curls (page 169). *Beginner:* 1 set of 3 to 10 reps, 3 days per week. *Intermediate:* 2 sets of 10 reps, 3 days per week.

Side-Lying Straight-Leg Raises (page 174). *Beginner:* 1 set of 3 to 10 reps with each leg, 3 days per week. *Intermediate:* 2 sets of 10 reps with each leg, 3 days per week.

Week 2

Inner-Leg Raises (page 176). *Beginner:* 1 set of 3 to 10 reps with each leg, 3 days per week. *Intermediate:* 2 sets of 10 reps with each leg, 3 days per week.

Prone Single-Leg Raises (page 170). *Beginner:* 1 set of 3 to 10 reps with each leg, 3 days per week. *Intermediate:* 2 sets of 10 reps with each leg, 3 days per week.

Leg Extensions (page 166). *Beginner:* 3 to 10 reps with each leg, 3 days per week. *Intermediate:* 2 sets of 10 reps with each leg, 3 days per week.

Week 3

Standing Abductions (page 175). *Beginner:* 1 set of 3 to 10 reps with each leg, 3 days per week. *Intermediate:* 2 sets of 10 reps with each leg, 3 days per week.

Pelvic Lifts (page 173). *Beginner:* 1 set of 10 reps, 3 days per week. *Intermediate:* 2 sets of 10 reps, 3 days per week.

Leg Curls (page 169). *Beginner:* 1 set of 3 to 10 reps, 3 days per week. *Intermediate:* 2 sets of 10 reps, 3 days per week.

Week 4

Leg Extensions (page 166). *Beginner:* 3 to 10 reps with each leg, 3 days per week. *Intermediate:* 2 sets of 10 reps with each leg, 3 days per week.

Inner-Leg Raises (page 176). *Beginner:* 1 set of 3 to 10 reps with each leg, 3 days per week. *Intermediate:* 2 sets of 10 reps with each leg, 3 days per week.

Pelvic Lifts (page 173). *Beginner:* 1 set of 10 reps, 3 days per week. *Intermediate:* 2 sets of 10 reps, 3 days per week.

Exercises: A 30-Day Intermediate Program

As you gain strength, switch to this program.

Week 1

Lunges (page 167). *Beginner:* 1 set of 3 to 10 reps with each leg, 3 days per week. *Intermediate:* 2 sets of 10 reps with each leg, 3 days per week.

Back-Leg Extensions (page 171). *Beginner:* 1 set of 3 to 10 reps with each leg, 3 days per week. *Intermediate:* 2 sets of 10 reps with each leg, 3 days per week.

Seated Inner-Leg Raises (page 177). *Beginner:* 1 set of 3 to 10 reps with each leg, 3 days per week. *Intermediate:* 2 sets of 10 reps with each leg, 3 days per week.

Week 2

Standing Abductions (page 175). *Beginner:* 1 set of 3 to 10 reps with each leg, 3 days per week. *Intermediate:* 2 sets of 10 reps with each leg, 3 days per week.

Lunges (page 167). *Beginner:* 1 set of 3 to 10 reps with each leg, 3 days per week. *Intermediate:* 2 sets of 10 reps with each leg, 3 days per week.

Bent-Leg Extensions (page 172). *Beginner:* 1 set of 3 to 10 reps with each leg, 3 days per week. *Intermediate:* 2 sets of 10 reps with each leg, 3 days per week.

Week 3

Butterfly-Leg Raises (page 178). *Beginner:* 1 set of 3 to 10 reps with each leg, 3 days per week. *Intermediate:* 2 sets of 10 reps with each leg, 3 days per week.

Lunges (page 167). *Beginner:* 1 set of 3 to 10 reps with each leg, 3 days per week. *Intermediate:* 2 sets of 10 reps with each leg, 3 days per week.

Standing Abductions (page 175). *Beginner:* 1 set of 3 to 10 reps with each leg, 3 days per week. *Intermediate:* 2 sets of 10 reps with each leg, 3 days per week.

Week 4

Pelvic Lifts (page 173). *Beginner:* 1 set of 10 reps, 3 days per week. *Intermediate:* 2 sets of 10 reps, 3 days per week.

Butterfly-Leg Raises (page 178). *Beginner:* 1 set of 3 to 10 reps with each leg, 3 days per week. *Intermediate:* 2 sets of 10 reps with each leg, 3 days per week.

Squats (page 168). *Beginner:* 3 to 10 reps, 3 days per week. *Intermediate:* 2 sets of 10 reps, 3 days per week.

Stretching into Shape

Stretching keeps your muscles flexible, helping to prepare them for exercise and recover from the effort afterward. Skip the stretches and you won't get nearly the benefits you should from aerobic exercise and resistance training.

"Stretching helps you move freely during aerobic exercise, it enables your muscles to build more strength during weight training, and it helps keep muscles long and lean," says Sharon Willett, a physical therapist and sports trainer at the Virginia Sportsmedicine Institute in Arlington, Virginia.

Stretching increases your range of motion by making your muscles, tendons, and joints more flexible. So the more you stretch, the greater benefit you'll get from your workouts, and the sooner you'll see results.

Experts agree you should warm up your muscles before stretching, to avoid tearing "cold" or stiff muscles.

Stretching Prevents Muscle Strain

Lack of flexibility not only slows your progress but also can lead to injury, which can derail even the best-laid exercise routines. And unless you've been athletic all your life, chances are you're not as flexible as you need to be to get the most out of your body-toning workouts.

"Aside from the aging process, our habits and daily activities can also cause our muscles and tendons to shorten," says Willett. Even your shoes can inhibit your flexibility. For example, wearing high heels shortens the hamstrings and calves. This won't be a problem when you're sitting still, says Willett. But if you try to do a leg curl or a squat, the shortened muscles won't do the job willingly. If you try to push a shortened muscle or tendon through too much exercise or range of motion, you'll develop pain or an injury, such as tendinitis (inflammation of the tendon).

Ironically, exercise, too, can affect flexibility. "Weight training and weight-bearing exercise like jogging contract muscles again and again, shortening the muscles and tendons involved," says Willett. "So you have to take the time to stretch out your muscles again after you use them. If you do so, your muscles and tendons will retain their elasticity and get even stronger. An exercise program that includes all three elements—cardiovascular, strength, and flexibility—will keep your muscles and tendons in the best shape possible."

In addition to keeping you flexible, stretching burns calories and helps you relax.

"Stretching isn't aerobic," concedes Willett. "But you'll burn more calories by stretching than you will by sitting and doing nothing." For a 150-pound woman, 30 minutes of stretching burns 60 to 100 calories—about the same as gentle yoga—compared with 22 calories for sitting still.

The Right Way to Stretch

Experts recommend that you stretch all your muscle groups, rather than just doing the stretches that target your particular trouble spot. All your muscles and tendons work together, so if you ignore one stretch, you won't get maximum benefit from the others. For maximum effectiveness, keep a few rules in mind when you stretch, says Willett.

Warm your muscles. Stretching is not a warmup. Spend at least 5 minutes doing some form of light aerobic exercise, such as walking, climbing stairs, or cleaning the house. Work hard enough so that you feel warm and sweat slightly. Then, if you stretch after your workout, your muscles will be warm and supple.

Don't bounce. Pushing your muscles in short, jerky movements tears the muscle fibers. Instead, slowly and evenly move into the stretch until you feel resistance, then back off a little and hold that position.

Hold each stretch for 20 seconds. "Stretches held for at least 20 seconds increase flexibility the most," says Willett. And don't hold your breath. Instead, take two or three deep breaths as you hold the stretch.

Do each stretch two, three, or four times. The real benefits come in increments, with each subsequent stretch.

When (and How Often) to Stretch

Stretching doesn't take much time—as little as 10 minutes should do it. And it's easy to fit into a busy workout schedule—all you need is an exercise mat. Use the exercises on pages 179 to 186 as the basis for your stretching routine. As for when to stretch, you have a number of options.

- If you've just begun your exercise program, it's best to stretch each muscle group immediately after an activity in which you've used those muscles, says Willett. So if you're doing squats to tone your butt, for example, stretch the gluteus muscles immediately after the exercise. And if you're working out every day, that means you'll stretch every day.

- If you're comfortable with your routine and never feel sore afterward, says Willett, feel free to do all of your stretches at the end of your workout.
- If it's convenient, you can also stretch without doing other exercise (except warming up). You'll benefit from two half-hour sessions a week even on days when you don't exercise.

"You can even stretch while you watch TV," says Willett. "There's no reason to be formal about it."

Curl-Ups 1

Muscles Worked
Upper abs

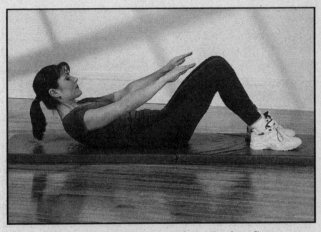

Lie on your back with your pelvis tilted to flatten your back against the floor, arms at your sides, knees bent at approximately a 90-degree angle, and your feet flat on the floor.

Using your upper abdominal muscles, raise your head and shoulders from the floor, as shown. Your arms should be extended out in front. Hold for 2 seconds. Then lower your shoulders to the floor in a slow, controlled motion, touching your shoulders lightly on the floor. Repeat.

Curl-Ups 2

Muscles Worked
Upper abs

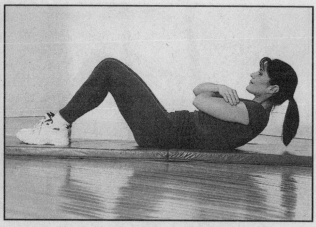

Lie on your back with your pelvis tilted to flatten your back, arms folded across your chest, knees bent approximately 90 degrees, and your feet flat on the floor.

Using your upper abdominal muscles, raise your head and shoulders from the floor toward your knees, as shown. Hold for 2 seconds. Then lower your upper body in a slow, controlled motion, touching your shoulders lightly on the floor. Repeat.

Knee-Up Crunches

Muscles Worked
Upper abs

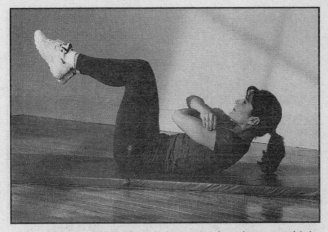

   Lie on your back with your legs raised so that your thighs are perpendicular to your body and your calves and feet are parallel to the floor. Fold your arms across your chest.

   Using the muscles of your upper abs, raise your shoulders and upper back off the floor in a forward curling motion, as shown. Hold for 2 seconds. Then slowly lower your shoulders to the starting position, lightly touching them to the floor. Repeat.

Hip Raises

Muscles Worked
Lower abs

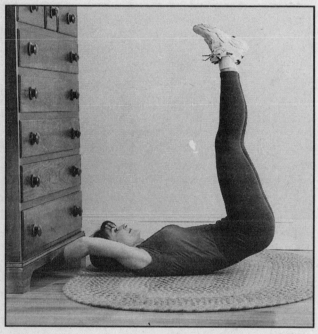

Lie on your back with your legs extended upward, toes pointed, and your arms extended overhead. Hold on to a heavy, secure piece of furniture such as the bottom of a desk, dresser, or couch.

Using your lower abdominal muscles, raise your hips off the floor and lift your legs, knees slightly flexed, straight in the air, as shown. Hold for 2 seconds. Then lower your legs, touching your hips lightly on the floor; repeat.

Modified Knee Raises

Muscles Worked
Lower abs

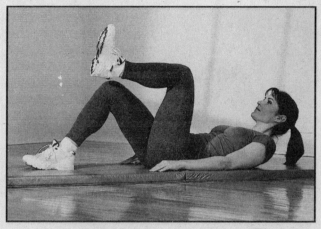

Lie on your back with your pelvis tilted to flatten your back and your knees bent. Your arms should be extended next to your body with your hands palms down, your head up, and your shoulder blades slightly off the floor.

Using your lower abdominals, raise one leg at a time toward your chest in a slow, controlled motion, as shown. Hold for 2 seconds. Then lower your leg slowly until your heel lightly touches the floor. Repeat with the opposite leg.

Pelvic Tilts

Muscles Worked
Lower abs

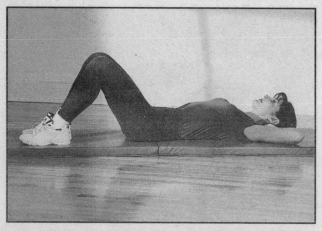

Lie flat on your back with your knees bent at approximately a 90-degree angle and your hands behind your head, elbows extended to your sides, and your head on the floor.

In a slow, controlled manner, lift your pelvis up and toward your rib cage, tightening your lower abdominal muscles and gently "pushing" your back into the floor. Hold for 2 seconds. Relax and let your pelvis rotate back to its normal position. Repeat.

Reverse Curls

Muscles Worked

Lower abs

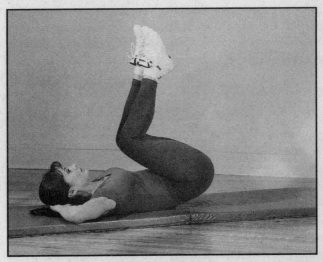

Lie flat on your back with your head on the floor, your hands behind your head supporting your neck, and your elbows out. Raise your legs so that your thighs are perpendicular to your body and your calves and feet are parallel to the floor.

Using your lower abs, raise your hips toward your rib cage, with your knees toward your forehead, as shown. Hold for a count of 2. Then lower your hips in a slow, controlled motion, keeping your abs contracted until your hips contact the floor. Repeat.

Diagonal Curl-Ups 1

Muscles Worked
Obliques

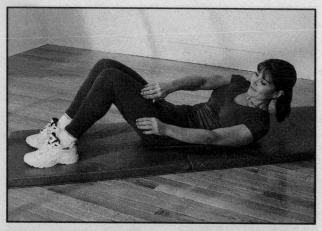

Lie on your back with your feet flat on the floor, your knees bent at approximately a 90-degree angle, your pelvis tilted to flatten your back, and your arms straight at your sides.

Extend your arms, as shown, and use your oblique muscles to raise your head and shoulders, rotating to one side as your shoulders lift off the floor. Hold for 2 seconds. Then lower your shoulders in a slow, controlled motion, touching them lightly to the floor. Repeat the exercise on the opposite side.

Diagonal Curl-Ups 2

Muscles Worked
Obliques

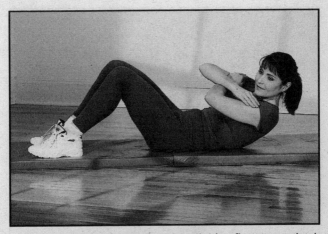

Lie on your back with your pelvis tilted to flatten your back against the floor, your knees bent at approximately a 90-degree angle, your feet flat on the floor, and your arms folded across your chest.

Use your oblique muscles to raise your head and shoulders from the floor, rotating to one side as your shoulders lift off the floor, as shown. Hold for 2 seconds. Lower your shoulders in a slow, controlled motion, touching them lightly to the floor. Repeat the exercise rotating in the opposite direction.

Side Bends

Muscles Worked
Obliques

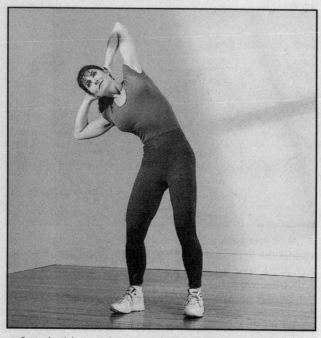

   Stand with your knees slightly bent, feet shoulder-width apart, hands behind your head, and elbows extended out.
   Using your oblique muscles, bend to your right side in a slow, controlled movement, bringing your right elbow toward your right knee, as shown. Return to the starting position. Repeat the movement to the same side until you have completed your repetitions, then perform the same exercise on the opposite side.

Side Jackknives

Muscles Worked
Obliques

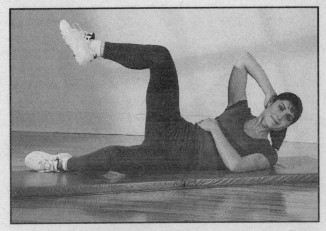

Lie on your left side with your legs together, your knees bent, and your thighs almost perpendicular to your body. Your left arm should be close to your body for support, with your left hand on your waist. Your right hand should be on the side of your head, with elbow bent.

Using your oblique muscles, raise your top leg while simultaneously raising your head, shoulders, and torso, as shown. Hold for 2 seconds. Then lower in a controlled motion. After completing your repetitions, repeat on the opposite side.

Leg Extensions

Muscles Worked
Quadriceps (fronts of thighs)

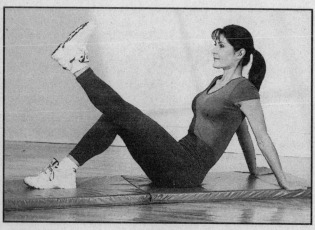

Supporting your trunk with your arms, sit on the floor with one leg extended, the knee slightly bent and foot flexed. Bend your opposite leg and place your foot flat on the floor.

Keeping your knee slightly bent and your foot flexed, lift your leg in a slow and controlled movement until your knee reaches the height of the knee of your bent leg, as shown. Return to the starting position. Repeat with the other leg when the set is completed.

Lunges

Muscles Worked

Quadriceps (fronts of thighs), gluteals (buttocks)

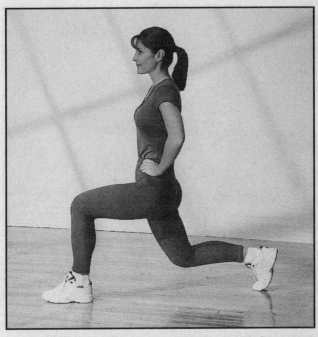

Stand with your feet about 6 inches apart and your toes pointed straight ahead, in their natural position. For balance, rest your hands on your hips.

Step forward with your left foot as far as possible, bending your right knee as you do. In a controlled move, continue the lunge until your right knee almost touches the floor, as shown, and then slowly return to the starting position. Do one set, then repeat with the opposite leg.

Squats

Muscles Worked

Quadriceps (fronts of thighs), gluteals (buttocks)

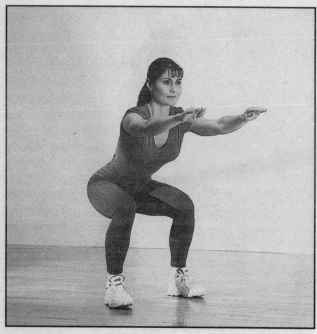

Stand with your feet shoulder-width apart. Tighten your abdomen and stand straight, looking directly ahead, focusing on a point so that your head and back are straight throughout the entire exercise.

Slowly lower yourself into a squatting position by bending your legs at the knees.

Descend to a position where your thighs are parallel to the ground, as shown. Return to the starting position. Repeat.

Leg Curls

Muscles Worked
Hamstrings (backs of thighs)

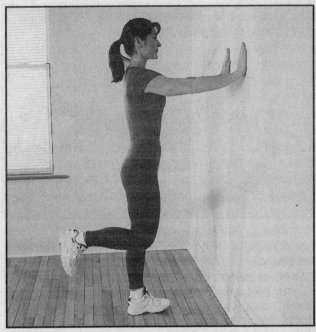

Stand facing a wall with your hands on the wall for balance and your feet approximately 12 to 15 inches from the wall.

Slowly bend one leg at the knee, raising the heel toward your buttocks in a slow, controlled movement until your lower leg is parallel to the floor, as shown, then return to the starting position. Do one set, then repeat with the opposite leg.

Prone Single-Leg Raises

Muscles Worked
Hamstrings (backs of thighs), gluteals (buttocks)

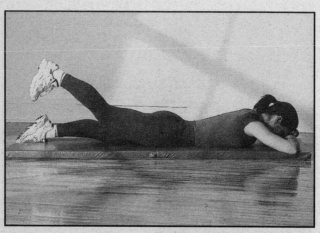

Lie flat on your stomach with your legs extended and your hands folded in front of you, with your forehead resting on your hands.

Keeping your leg extended, your foot flexed, and your knee slightly bent, raise one leg in a slow, controlled motion (as shown) until you feel tightness in the muscles of your buttocks. Return to the starting position. Complete one set, then repeat with the other leg.

Back-Leg Extensions

Muscles Worked

Hamstrings (backs of thighs), gluteals (buttocks)

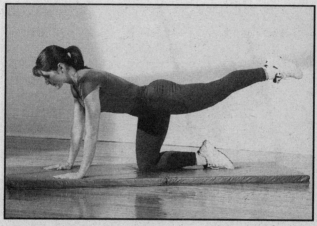

Get down on all fours, with your arms fully extended, elbows locked, and your head and neck aligned with your spine.

Using your buttocks muscles, extend and raise one leg until your thigh is parallel to the floor, as shown. Return to the starting position. Do one set, then repeat with the opposite leg.

Bent-Leg Extensions

Muscles Worked

Hamstrings (backs of thighs), gluteals (buttocks)

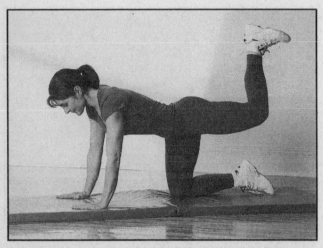

Get down on all fours, with your arms fully extended, elbows locked, and your head and neck aligned with your spine.

Extend one leg, bent at a 90-degree angle, with your foot flexed, until your thigh is parallel to the ground, as shown. Return to the starting position. Do one set, then repeat with your other leg.

Pelvic Lifts

Muscles Worked
Hamstrings (backs of thighs), gluteals (buttocks)

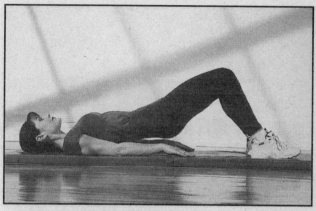

Lie on your back with your knees bent and your feet flat on the floor, with your hands at your sides, palms down.

Lift your pelvis toward the ceiling, as shown, squeezing your buttocks, until your back is straight. Repeat.

Side-Lying Straight-Leg Raises

Muscles Worked

Gluteals (buttocks), abductors (outer thighs)

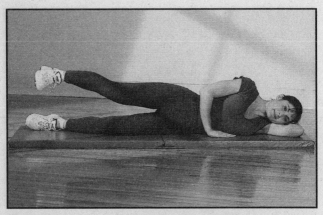

Lie on your side with your legs together, supporting your head with one arm and balancing yourself with the other.

Keeping your upper leg rotated in (toe pointing down) and your foot flexed, raise the top leg in a slow, controlled motion approximately 10 to 12 inches off the floor (as shown) without moving your torso. Return to the starting position. Do one set, then repeat with the opposite leg.

Standing Abductions

Muscles Worked
Gluteals (buttocks), abductors (outer thighs)

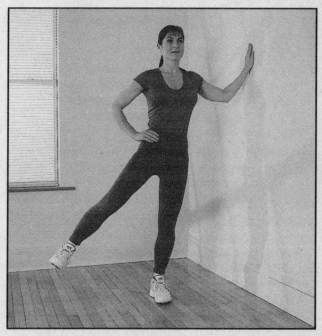

Holding on to a wall for balance, stand with your knees slightly bent.

Keeping your knee slightly bent, lift the working leg to the side, as shown. Your foot should be flexed. Lift as far as you can without moving your upper torso. Return to the starting position. Do one set, then repeat with the opposite leg.

Inner-Leg Raises

Muscles Worked

Adductors (inner thighs)

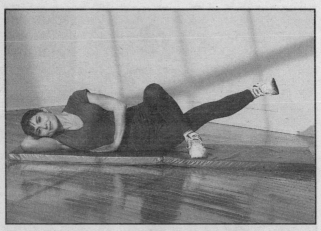

Lie on your side, supporting your head with your arm and your upper body with your opposite hand. Bend your top leg and place it in front of your other leg so your foot is flat on the floor and your bottom leg is straight with the knee slightly bent and the foot flexed.

Raise your bottom leg as high as possible without moving the rest of your body, as shown. Return to the starting position without touching your foot to the floor. Do one set, then repeat with your other leg.

Seated Inner-Leg Raises

Muscles Worked
Adductors (inner thighs)

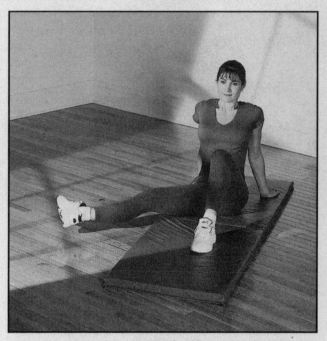

Sit with one leg bent and the foot flat on the floor, leaning back and supporting yourself. Extend the other leg, bending your knee slightly, flexing your foot, and rotating your hip (toes pointed out).

Move the working leg outward as far as you can without losing your balance, as shown. Return to the starting position without touching your foot to the floor. Do one set, then repeat with your other leg.

Butterfly-Leg Raises

Muscles Worked

Adductors (inner thighs)

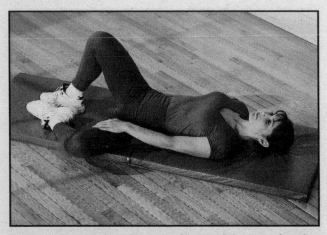

Lie on your back with one leg bent and the same foot flat on the floor. The other leg should be bent and lowered to the side. The sole of the foot of the lowered leg should face the side of the other foot.

Keeping your legs bent, raise the lowered knee toward the opposite knee, pressing against the inner thigh with your hand, as shown, for resistance. Return to the starting position. Do one set, then repeat with the other leg.

Press-Ups

Muscles Stretched
Upper and lower abs

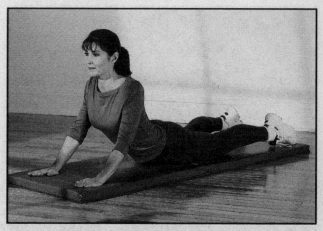

Lie on your stomach with your hands on the floor, directly under your shoulders. Raise your upper body as far as you can by straightening your elbows and arching your back, keeping your hips in contact with the floor, as shown. Keep your chest upright so your shoulders are not hunched up by your ears. You should feel the stretch along the front of your body. You can lift your chin, but don't drop your head back. Hold for 20 to 30 seconds. Repeat four times.

Spinal Twists

Muscles Stretched

Middle- and lower-back muscles

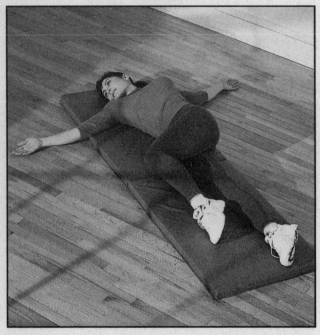

Lie on your back with your arms out to each side (perpendicular to your body). Keeping your shoulders flat on the floor, bend your left knee up toward your chest and slowly bring the bent leg across your body, as shown. Turn your head to look at your right hand until you feel a stretch. Hold for 20 to 30 seconds, then repeat to the other side. Do four stretches on each side.

Figure-Four Stretches

Muscles Stretched
Gluteus maximus (buttocks)

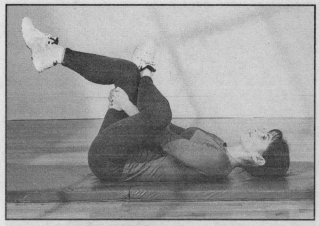

Lie on your back with both knees bent. Cross your left foot over your right knee. Place your hands behind your right knee and slowly bring your knee toward your chest, as shown. You should feel the stretch in your left buttock area. Hold for 20 to 30 seconds, then repeat on the opposite side. Stretch each side four times.

Hip Flexor Stretches

Muscles Stretched
Muscles in front of the hips and thighs

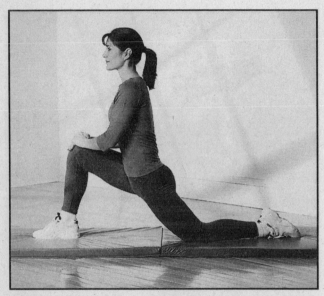

Begin by kneeling on the floor. Bring your right knee in front of you and place your foot flat on the floor. Your left knee should be resting on the floor. Slowly lean forward to extend your left leg back, keeping your shin and knee on the floor, as shown. You should feel a stretch in the front of your right hip and thigh. Make sure your right knee isn't extending farther than your toes. Hold this stretch for 20 to 30 seconds, then switch sides. Repeat four times.

Hip/Quad Stretches

Muscle Stretched

Iliotibial band (outside of legs from hips to knees) and quadriceps

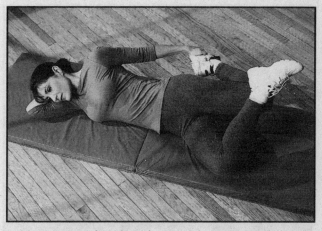

Lie on your right side with your right arm extended under your head. Bend your left knee and use your left hand to pull your heel up toward your buttock. Take your right foot and place it on top of your left knee, as shown. Apply a downward pressure with your right foot, pushing your left knee toward the floor. Hold for 20 to 30 seconds and then repeat on the opposite side. Repeat the stretch four times on each side.

Inner-Thigh and Groin Stretches

Muscles Worked
Inner thighs and groin

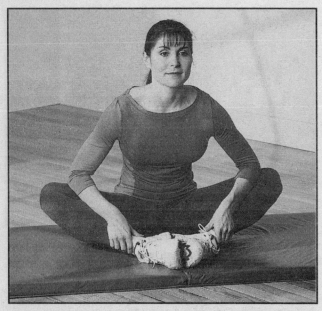

Sit on the floor with your back straight. Place the heels of your feet together and drop your knees out to your sides. Clasp your hands around your ankles, as shown. Using your forearms, slowly press your knees toward the floor until you feel a stretch. Do not force your knees to the floor. Hold for 20 to 30 seconds. Repeat four times.

Hamstring Stretches

Muscles Stretched
Backs of thighs

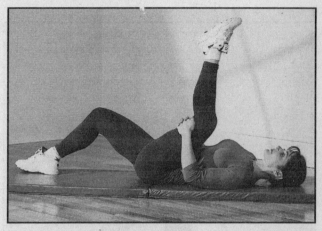

Lie on your back, keeping your lower back pressed to the floor. Bend both knees and keep your feet flat on the floor. Bring your hands to the back of your left thigh, and slowly straighten and raise your left leg. Gently pull your leg in toward your torso (as shown) until you feel a stretch in the back of your leg. Hold for 20 to 30 seconds, then repeat with the other leg. Repeat four times with each leg. As this stretch becomes easier, keep the resting leg straight out in front of you, instead of bent, for more of a stretch.

Calf Stretches

Muscles Stretched

Gastrocnemius and soleus (backs and sides of calves) and Achilles tendon

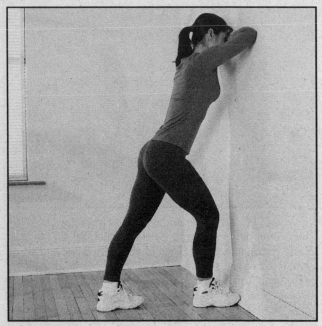

Stand with your forearms against a wall and your right leg out in front of you with the knee bent. Your knees shouldn't extend past your toes. Keep your left leg straight and your feet flat on the floor. Slowly lean forward on your right leg, as shown, until you feel a stretch in the back of your calf. Hold for 20 to 30 seconds. This will stretch the upper part of the calf. Then slightly bend your left knee and repeat to stretch the lower part of the calf. Hold each stretch for 20 to 30 seconds, then switch sides. Repeat four times with each leg.

PART FOUR

The Best Fat-Burning Exercises

13 Ways to Work Off Fat and Calories

Thanks to a daily aerobic workout that consisted of walking (coupled with a small amount of weight training), Barbara Evanson lost 23 inches, mostly from her waist, abdomen, and hips.

"I am quite overweight and have a long way to go," says Barbara, 51, a certified nursing assistant who lives in Cadott, Wisconsin. "But I can't believe I started to see changes in just one month! Even my energy level is higher. When I want a change of pace from walking, I spend 1 to 2 hours at a time weeding my garden."

As Barbara's success story proves, working out aerobically doesn't mean you have to run or join an aerobics class to lose weight and shape up. Everyday activities like walking and gardening count. They can and do burn fat and calories—just like more strenuous workouts—and can help you flatten your abs, trim your thighs, and tuck your butt.

Jump-Starting Your Metabolism

Aerobic activities are big calorie burners, and—along with a diet that controls fat and calories—they go a long way toward burning away excess weight. One reason: They speed your metabolism. When you work out hard enough to raise your heart rate, it increases your metabolism during the exercise, burning more calories. Eventually, it may increase your metabolic rate, the rate at which you burn calories as you go about your daily business. Metabolic changes, in turn, improve your body's ability to burn fat and make your muscles better able to use oxygen for this purpose. As your level of aerobic fitness increases, your heart, lungs, and muscles become more efficient, so you can do more without getting tired.

Once you become more physically active, people may start noticing that you look thinner and more muscular. Most aerobic activity doesn't build muscle, but your muscles will look more toned, and you'll lose fat, giving you a leaner look overall. For that reason, you'll probably notice that your clothes fit better before you actually see your weight change on the scale.

Looking good isn't the only benefit to shaking your tail feather. You'll feel good, too. Evidence shows that participating in aerobic exercise can help reduce symptoms of depression and anxiety and make you feel generally better emotionally. A study conducted by the department of human performance and health promotion at the University of New Orleans, for example, found that 36 women and 6 men who enrolled in step aerobics classes of varying intensity felt less tense, depressed, fatigued, and angry after the more intense workouts than they did after the less intense workouts.

Some experts say that exercise elevates your mood simply by freeing your mind from everyday concerns. "It may be just that you're having fun," suggests Charles Corbin, Ph.D., professor in the department of exercise science and physical education at Arizona State University in Tempe. "You're doing something you like." Given that many women blame unwanted weight gain, in part, on a tendency to overeat when they're tired, bored, tense, or angry, the psychological benefits of aerobic exercise can play a part in your success.

Another possible explanation for why exercise elevates mood: Some experts say that during and after exercise, your brain releases endorphins, chemical substances associated with pleasure. You've probably heard athletes or others refer to this as an endorphin high. But everyday exercisers like you can enjoy the same uplifting effect.

How Hard Do You Have to Work?

To reap the basic health benefits of aerobic exercise, you need to work at an intensity that raises your heart rate, and you need to do this for a total of at least 30 minutes a day, three to five times a week.

If you're aiming to lose weight, you need to exercise aerobically at a moderate intensity for 30 to 60 minutes most days of the week. "Thirty minutes is the point at which fat is being used as the primary energy source," says Laurie L. Tis, Ph.D., associate professor in the department of kinesiology and health at Georgia State University in Atlanta.

How do you know what's moderate intensity? One way is to calculate your target heart rate. To do this, subtract your age from 220. This tells you your approximate maximum heart rate. You don't want to work at your maximum. Instead, you need to calculate your target heart rate zone—a range, depending on your fitness level, that's 60 to 90 percent of your maximum. To do that, multiply your maximum rate by 0.6 if you want to exercise at 60 percent of your maximum (low intensity), which is good for beginners, 0.7 for 70 percent of your maximum (moderate intensity), or 0.8 for 80 percent (high intensity).

This isn't as hard as it sounds. To calculate her target heart rate zone, a 52-year-old woman would subtract 52 from 220 for her maximum heart rate of 168. To work out at 70 percent of this maximum rate, she would multiply 168 by 0.7, for a target heart rate of 118.

You can make sure your heart rate falls within your target range while you exercise by checking your pulse. Place two or three fingers lightly in the inside of your opposite wrist below the base of your thumb. Count the beats for 1 minute to get the pulse rate, which is the beat of the heart as felt through the walls of the arteries. Alternatively, you can count your pulse for 15 seconds and multiply by four.

Experts say that if you're new to aerobic exercise, you can aim for a target heart rate of 60 percent of your maximum. Once you're in pretty good shape, you can work up to 90 percent.

If you have no patience with numbers, there are a few other, simpler ways to tell if you're exercising hard enough, says Michael Youssouf, a certified trainer and manager of trainer education and advancement at the Sports Center at Chelsea Piers in New York City. You're doing fine if you're breathing hard but not so hard that you can't carry on a conversation. Or if you've broken a sweat. Or you simply *feel* like you're working.

Want another way to rate intensity? Ask yourself how much longer you can carry on the activity. The activity should take enough out of you that you wouldn't be able to continue for hours, but you shouldn't be working so hard that you need to stop right away, says Youssouf.

As you continue to get in shape, what used to be strenuous becomes easier, so you must add to the duration, intensity, or frequency of the exercise or start doing a different, more challenging activity, says Youssouf.

Work Hard (But Not Too Hard)

Just as one-size-fits-all clothing tends not to fit any woman well, a strict and uncompromising exercise routine is uncomfortable for most individuals. All a woman needs to do is find some activities that allow her to work within a range that gets her heart pumping. In researching this book, we talked to dozens of women, each of whom tamed her trouble spots by doing something different. Some walked off the unwanted bulges. Some took up inline skating. Others found weight-loss nirvana on "new" equipment like elliptical trainers. Others turned to old standbys like stationary bicycles and cross-country ski machines.

For them, like many women, the key to sticking with an aerobic exercise program was to make it fun or interesting. "A lot of times, it's just a matter of finding an activity that you like," says Dr. Tis. "If you don't like walking, then try biking, mountain biking, or inline skating." Better still, try a mix of activities. Maybe on Mondays you play tennis, Wednesdays you attend an aerobics class, and Fridays you go bicycling with your family.

Only you can decide what works best for you. For some women, sticking with one form of exercise rather than doing a mix is best because they like to excel at one thing, says Martin Hoffman, M.D., professor in the department of physical medicine and rehabilitation at the Medical College of Wisconsin and director of the sports performance and technology laboratory, both in Milwaukee. So, for example, if you enjoy running, you may be motivated to do just this exercise by constantly trying to improve the time or distance of your runs. As you shop for an aerobic activity that suits your purposes, you'll also learn how to maximize the body-shaping benefits by maximizing your effort or frequency.

Another time-honored approach for women just beginning an exercise program—and one that works—is to find an exercise buddy, says Dr. Hoffman. "If you know that your friend is going to be there at six in the morning to go for a walk with you, you won't decide you're too tired today and sleep in."

By simply walking 30 minutes a day at a moderate pace, you will lose 5 to 15 pounds after 1 year, depending on your size, says Dr. Corbin. "The best form of exercise for weight control is the kind of exercise you will actually do," he adds.

Exercise or other physical activity can also become a time to maintain or strengthen family ties or friendships, says Dr. Tis. Go cycling with your kids and use the time not only to burn calories but also to talk to them. Or take your husband along on your evening walks and make the most of this time to yourselves.

Dr. Tis exercises regularly with one of her colleagues, "and it's our talk time. We work out and have 30 minutes away from the phones and the office and are able to just talk."

Getting Started

Before you start an aerobic exercise program, ask your doctor for advice if you answer yes to two or more of the following.

- You are over the age of 45.
- You are less than 55 and past menopause and not taking estrogen replacement therapy (which protects your heart).

- You smoke cigarettes.
- You have or have ever had high blood pressure or high cholesterol.
- You're sedentary—that is, you work at a desk, have no physically active hobbies or pastimes, or don't currently exercise regularly.
- You have a family history of heart disease, high blood pressure, or high cholesterol.

If your foray into fitness takes you to a health club or other group setting, don't be intimidated by how other women look or whether they are more proficient on treadmills, stairclimbers, or various other exercise machines, advises Dr. Tis.

"It's been my experience that if you can get through some of those initial insecurities, you'll be surprised at how exercise boosts your self-esteem," Dr. Tis says. "Just remember, you are there to improve *your* health and well-being. You want to feel good now and 25 years from now. So this is a commitment to yourself. You will feel more comfortable, and everything will start to fall into place."

Start by gently warming up: Walk at an easy pace for 5 minutes to get your blood circulating. Then do some gentle stretches (no bouncing) before you start your aerobic activity. When you've ended your activity, allow your body to cool down. Walk for about 3 to 5 minutes. Then do some gentle stretches, which will help increase or maintain flexibility, says Dr. Tis.

When starting out, don't be discouraged if you can do only, say, 10 minutes on a particular exercise, cautions Dr. Tis. Instead, just lighten the tension on the machine the next time, or ease the pace, and try for 15 minutes. Then try to build upon that gradually.

"This isn't a competition or a race," points out Dr. Tis. "You have to stay within your abilities so it's comfortable."

How much should you increase your performance before leveling off for a while? "The rule of thumb is 10 percent per week," says Dr. Tis. "That's probably a little low. The thing to remember is that you can increase the intensity, increase the time, or increase the resistance on some of the machines, but do only one increase a week."

For example, say that you're walking at 3 miles per hour on a treadmill for 20 minutes at a time. You're cruisin'— hardly huffing, scarcely sweating. Here are your options: You can increase your time on the machine to 22 to 23 minutes. Or you can stay at 20 minutes but increase your speed to 3½ to 4 miles per hour. Or you can do neither but steepen the degree of incline.

"If you are really enjoying working out, you could keep the intensity and duration the same but add an extra day. And remember, take one day off a week, no matter how fit you are.

No matter which method you choose, you'll be on your way toward the body you desire.

To banish your extra weight and tone trouble spots like your belly, butt, and thighs, you can choose from more than a dozen types of fat-burning activities, like walking or bicycling, inline skating or jumping rope. In the pages that follow are descriptions of 13 popular exercises.

Bicycling

You say the last time you rode a bike, it was a pink two-wheeler with a banana seat and streamers hanging off the handlebars? Well, you've grown up, and so has the bicycling industry. According to the National Sporting Goods Association, 45 percent of all adult bike riders are women. And more and more bikes are designed for women. No, women's bikes don't have pink paint and streamers. But they do have seats and frames designed for the female anatomy. And they're sturdy and easy to ride—even if you've never been on a bike in your life.

"If your knees, ankles, or hips bother you when you walk, then cycling might be a great, pain-free way to exercise and lose weight," says Edmund Burke, Ph.D., professor of exercise science at the University of Colorado in Colorado Springs and coauthor of *Fitness Cycling*. "Unlike walking or running, cycling isn't a weight-bearing exercise—the bicycle, not your bones and joints, supports your weight."

Body-Shaping Benefits

"The body-shaping benefits of cycling are primarily from the hips down," says Dr. Burke. "Bicycling works the muscles in your buttocks, front and back thighs, and lower legs." These are the largest muscles in your body, and when you use them to perform high-intensity work, such as cycling, you burn a lot of calories. (Remember, calories are a form of energy, and it takes energy to do physical work.) So if you bicycle regularly:

- You'll strengthen and tone the muscles of your lower body during your workout.
- You'll burn off a fair number of stored calories—or fat.
- You'll burn 130 to 345 calories per half-hour, depending on your speed and terrain, if you weigh 150 pounds.

Psychological Benefits

If you're like a lot of women, you probably have wonderful memories of exploring your neighborhood by bike as a kid, riding with your friends for hours. Yet somewhere along the way toward adulthood—probably once you got your driver's license—your bike started to gather dust in the garage, becoming a forgotten relic of the past. And that's a shame.

"You'll enjoy riding a bike as an adult just as much as you did as a kid," says Dr. Burke. "Bicycling gets you outside just like walking does, but it expands your terrain. When you get on a bike, you can see more of the world."

If you typically walk an hour a day for exercise and cover 3 to 4 miles, you can cycle for the same amount of time and cover 10 miles.

The Right Footwear

Unless you're competing in the world-famous, multi-day Tour de France bike race, you can cycle in comfortable, lightweight sneakers, as long as the soles have enough grip to stay put on the bike pedals, says Dr. Burke.

"Be sure to tuck the laces under the tongues of your shoes, though, so the laces don't get tangled in the pedals, chain, or chain guard," he adds.

Also, don't tie your laces too tightly or your feet will fall asleep while you ride. To keep your feet comfortable, choose socks made of blends of cotton and synthetic fibers like polypropylene, which wick away moisture and let your skin breathe.

What Else You'll Need

Aside from the right footwear, you'll need a bike and a helmet—both of which you should purchase at a bike shop where they sell and service bikes. Even if you have an old Schwinn you want to resurrect, you need to take it over to a bike shop for a tune-up before you head out down the driveway. It's almost sure to need new tires and some oil to lubricate the chains and gears.

"Bike shop owners know which bikes are good for beginners," says Dr. Burke. Bike shops usually work in tandem with their customers to keep their bikes working well, which means you'll be safer and your bike will last longer.

If you need a bike, you can choose from three types.

- Road bike. This bike looks like a 10-speed, which you may have ridden as a teenager. It has drop handlebars (they curve under) and smooth, narrow tires. These bikes are designed for speed, not comfort.
- Mountain bike. These bikes have flat handlebars (they don't curve) and fatter tires than road bikes. It's easier to balance on them. The tires are knobby, for better traction. They're designed for riding on un-

paved trails, over rocks and roots and such—but they function well on paved paths, too.

- Hybrid bike. These bikes have gears, handlebars, and frames similar to mountain bikes but with narrower tires for the smooth ride of a road bike. Experts tend to recommend hybrid bikes for adult women interested in bicycling.

"Hybrids generally have sturdier frames than road bikes, so they provide lots of stability," says Tim Blumenthal, executive director of the International Mountain Bicycling Association in Boulder, Colorado. "They're easy to ride on pavement. And if you want to ride in parks, hybrids can handle dirt trails and unpaved roads."

The right fit. Experts at bike shops are better equipped to measure you and your new equipment properly than salespeople at a department store. Ask for a bike designed especially for women. These have a steeper seat tube (the vertical tube) to position you correctly and a shorter top tube (running from the seat tube to the head tube and handlebars) to accommodate women's shorter torsos and arms. Or they may steer you toward a man's bike that the specialists reconfigure to fit you (moving handlebars or changing the seat, for instance, so you don't have to reach as far for the handlebars).

Proper fit is essential. "If your bike doesn't fit you properly, it will be too uncomfortable for you to ride regularly," says Dr. Burke. If you're not experienced at riding a bike with multiple gears, you may want to consider a bike with gears that are clearly numbered, to help you learn how to shift.

A comfortable seat. If you're serious about getting in shape, you'll be spending a fair amount of time in the saddle. So whichever style of bike you choose, you also need to feel comfortable in the saddle.

"You have to find a good bike with a comfortable seat, or else you'll be putting pressure on parts of your body that don't respond well to intense friction and excess weight," says Dr. Burke. So by all means, ask about special seats made for women. Some feature a wider back and a narrower, cutout nose that takes the weight off delicate tissues for a more comfortable ride. Others use a soft material on the underside, with less bracing (used for stiffness), than seats for men's bikes so that the saddle flexes to absorb impact.

A helmet. When you cycle outdoors, you must always wear a helmet to protect your head from impact if you collide with the pavement (or anything else). Many helmets are specially designed for women—a big help if, for example, you want to pull your hair back in a ponytail when you ride. Helmets sold in bike shops are almost always of equal quality because all are made to the same safety specifications. Further, the Consumer Product Safety Commission requires all helmets made or sold in the United States to meet federal safety standards. Consider a helmet with a vent to help keep you cool and those with reflective stripes and removable visors for riding at night and in the sun. Plan to wear a cap under your helmet only if the helmet is designed to accommodate a hat—otherwise, you compromise fit and safety.

Getting Started

Once you have a well-oiled bicycle that suits you to a T, it's time to head out into the wide world of road cycling.

Get to know your bike. Before taking off on a 10-mile trek, ride around your neighborhood or an empty parking lot to get to know the gears and brakes on your new equipment.

Practice shifting gears. "Most people who are new to biking keep their bikes in one gear because they aren't sure how to shift and haven't taken the time to get to know which gears will help them on which terrain," notes Dr. Burke.

Technically, the best way to figure out whether you're using the right gear for a specific terrain is to count your pedal strokes. To do this, count your pedal revolutions (on one leg) for 15 seconds, then multiply that number by four. Efficient riders do 80 to 100 revolutions per minute on flat roads and about 60 to 85 revolutions on hills. But for beginners, pedaling and counting while looking at your watch and trying to see where you're going is a bit tricky. An easier rule of thumb: Use the lower (smaller) gears on steeper terrain and the higher (larger) gears on flatter terrain. Then practice until you get a feel for the combination that enables you to pedal the most efficiently. If you're struggling, shift to an easier gear. If the wheels are spinning with little or no resistance, shift to a harder gear.

"Don't be afraid to play with your bike in the beginning," says Dr. Burke.

Experiment with hand positions. Some hand positions feel better than others. You might feel comfortable riding with your hands close together, while another bicyclist might prefer grasping the very edges of the handlebars.

Follow through when you pedal. Good pedaling involves technique. You have to use your leg muscles on the back end of the pedaling stroke—that is, when you're bringing the pedal back up and bending your leg—to pedal efficiently. To do this, just imagine that you're scraping mud from the bottom of your shoe. In other words, press your leg down, apply force when your foot is at the bottom of the stroke, then use your leg muscles to pull the bottom of your leg back up toward your butt, says Dr. Burke.

Lean forward—or stand—when going up hills. As you progress and begin to feel more comfortable on your bike, you'll spend more time out of the saddle. For instance, when you go into a turn, you'll lean forward, out of the seat. When you go up hills, you'll stand in order to get more power to your legs.

Watch out for cars, both moving and parked. If you ride on roads and streets, you probably know enough to pay attention to moving vehicles. But you also need to be aware of parked cars. Many street accidents take place when someone who has just parked her car opens the door straight into the path of a bike rider. "It takes practice to learn how to ride on crowded roads," cautions Blumenthal. "You should ride with traffic, not against it. Keep your eyes and ears open; both are important." That means no Walkman.

Take a lesson. Many bike shops offer clinics and classes for novice riders. You'll learn, for example, that as with driving a car, it's usually best to brake before a turn, rather than during one.

Cross-Country Ski Machines

Even if you live in sultry Miami, you can cross-country ski—on a ski simulator machine. These gizmos approximate the sliding-and-gliding motion of traversing snowy trails.

And what a workout!

"I just feel it's the best workout of any," says Jodi Paul, racquetball program director at the Allentown Racquetball and Fitness Club in Allentown, Pennsylvania. "You use your upper and lower body at the same time, whereas most equipment uses one or the other." Paul has owned a cross-country ski simulator for 8 years, swears by it, and teaches members of her club how to use the machine.

Body-Shaping Benefits

Here's what experts say you can expect if you use a cross-country ski machine as part of your body-shaping program.

- You'll get an all-around workout that works both your upper and your lower body, raising your heart rate more and burning more calories than if you used exercise equipment that works just one or the other.

- You'll work all your main muscles—quadriceps, hamstrings, hips, and glutes—as well as your back, arms, and shoulders.
- You'll burn 254 to 339 calories per half-hour, depending on intensity, if you weigh 150 pounds.

Psychological Benefits

As with other forms of exercise, women using cross-country ski machines can benefit emotionally, says Martin Hoffman, M.D., professor in the department of physical medicine and rehabilitation at the Medical College of Wisconsin and director of the sports performance and technology laboratory, both in Milwaukee. The rhythmic motion and the solitary nature of the exercise can be peaceful. Cross-country ski simulators take practice, though, so be patient. The psychological benefits don't kick in until you master the machine. First, concentrate on proper technique.

The Right Footwear

Unlike outdoor skiing, you needn't concern yourself with boots and bindings. Your feet will be inside toe cups on the machine, so you need only wear a pair of comfortable cross-trainers or running shoes. Paul prefers running shoes because their pointier toes fit more snugly in the footholds.

What Else You'll Need

If you're buying a cross-country ski machine for your home, you need to have a roomy area in which to use it.

On most models, the skis extend beyond the simulator—figure on an overall length of about 8 feet and a width of about 3 feet.

Other machines are shuffle-type skiers that don't extend beyond the machine's body. But some users insist

A Hard Machine Made Easier

A cross-country ski simulator gives a great full-body workout, but it's a tough piece of exercise equipment to master. To make working out easier while maximizing the benefits, follow these suggestions from experts.

Create tension. When you begin on the machine, make sure that there is some leg tension, even if it's only on the lowest setting. Otherwise, your feet may slide back too easily.

Set the rhythm. The hardest thing to learn on this machine is how to develop a rhythm in which your arms and legs are moving in conjunction, not at odds with each other. Try perfecting just your leg movements at first, resting your hands on the handlebars or bumper pad in front of you until you do. Then gradually begin coordinating arm motion and leg motion.

Position your legs. As you begin the lower-body movement, keep one foot forward and one back as though you're walking, rather than side by side.

Bend your knees, please. You should have "soft"—slightly bent—knees when you're using this machine.

Go all the way. Practice a full range of motion with your arms and legs when skiing in your home or gym.

Perfect your posture. Don't lean forward on the ski simulator. You should stand upright. If you rest your stomach on the bumper pad in front of you, you may be propelled off the back of the simulator.

these don't really simulate cross-country skiing, says Paul. "Still, they give a good workout and may be worth a look if space is a consideration."

Since fewer and fewer manufacturers are selling cross-country ski machines, most likely you'll be using a machine at a gym or fitness center. Either way, here's what to look for when choosing one.

Consider the design. Ski machines come in two basic types. One, called a dependent system, links the skis with poles that you move back and forth or up and down with your hands. One foot moves forward, and the other automatically moves back. These machines are easy and safe to use, but they aren't as challenging as independent systems and may become boring.

An independent system works each foot separately and uses a cable, rather than poles, that you pull with your hands. This type of machine takes longer to learn, but the independent foot action is smoother and more enjoyable to use. Also, an independent machine forces you to use your upper body, so it gives you a more balanced workout.

Check the machine's features. Your ski simulator should be sturdy and have separate resistance settings for the legs and arms so that you can increase the tension on either or both as you become more proficient in the use of the machine. It also should have a mechanism to adjust for arm length. This will enable you to use the machine comfortably regardless of your height. Some machines have electronic monitors that tell you how fast you're moving, how many calories you're burning, how long you've been on the machine, and how far you've traveled.

Get more, pay more. If you find a store that sells cross-country ski simulators, be aware that they go for about $450 or more. Don't buy the bargain-basement machines. "Those aren't even worth considering," says Dr. Hoffman.

Getting Started

Ski simulators are hard to get the hang of, but enthusiasts say they are worth the effort. Establishing a rhythm while moving your arms and legs is difficult.

"There's a big learning curve," says Laurie L. Tis, Ph.D., associate professor in the department of kinesiology and health at Georgia State University in Atlanta. "It takes practice."

Master the leg action first. To speed up the learning process, work on the leg motion alone, then practice the arm action by itself, before trying the two movements together.

Warm up your legs. Warm up for 5 to 10 minutes before a workout on a ski simulator, recommends Dr. Tis. Start out at a leisurely walking pace for a few minutes, then gradually increase the speed or resistance for a few minutes and let this serve as your warmup. Doing so will help you avoid strain and injury.

Give it time. Don't be discouraged if the machine initially feels as strange as dancing on a water bed. "For most people, their first time on is not the time to judge whether they are going to like it or not," says Dr. Hoffman. If you're considering buying a machine, he recommends trying one out at your local Y or fitness center several times before making a purchase.

Elliptical Training

An elliptical trainer is about as close as anything comes to a perfect exercise machine. It looks like a combination treadmill, cross-country ski machine, and stepping machine, and it combines the movements (and benefits) of hiking, cross-country skiing, and biking. Working out on the trainer feels like standing on a cross-country ski machine, but instead of your feet moving back and forth, the machine forces them to move around in an oval (or elliptical) pattern.

Using the elliptical trainer doesn't create any impact, so it's easy on your joints. And it's versatile: You can use it to climb or glide. For your effort, you'll get a calorie-burning workout that pumps your heart like an all-out run without the same stress and strain on the joints in your body—the ideal workout routine for overweight women who don't have the wherewithal to jog. Even though most women burn hundreds of calories on the elliptical machine, they feel as if they're just strolling along. As a result, you can get rid of unwanted accumulations of fat on your belly, butt, or thighs without having to push yourself as hard as you do on other machines.

"We compared 16 men and women, each of whom used an elliptical trainer, a treadmill, an exercise bike, and a stair stepper," says John Porcari, Ph.D., professor of exercise and sports science at the University of Wisconsin–La Crosse. "Even if you use the elliptical trainer at the same intensity as running on the treadmill, the impact is the same as walking, so it puts less stress on your feet and legs. You get the same workout as running, with only half the potential for injuries. It's an outstanding piece of equipment."

Body-Shaping Benefits

Here's what you can expect when you use an elliptical trainer regularly.

- When you move forward on the machine, you'll work your quadriceps (the big muscles on the front of your thighs) and gluteus muscles (which shape your backside).
- You'll tone and slim your entire lower body.
- You'll notice that your legs are shapelier than ever because elliptical training uses all the muscles of the legs, large and small.
- You'll burn approximately 10 calories per minute while you work.

Psychological Benefits

If you've tried treadmill running and found it boring or if you're ready for a change, an elliptical trainer offers varied programs to keep you moving for a long time to come. Most converts find they love elliptical trainers simply because they're so easy to use, says Dr. Porcari.

The Right Footwear

Because your feet don't leave the elliptical trainer's surface, any lightweight athletic shoe will suffice, says Gregory Florez, owner of Fitness First, a personal training company in Chicago and Salt Lake City. Just be sure not to tie the laces too tightly or your feet will start to feel numb.

To keep your feet dry and blister-free, pair those shoes up with athletic wear socks of synthetic or cotton/synthetic fiber blends that "breathe," advises Florez.

What Else You'll Need

An elliptical trainer has various settings: resistance, speed, and, usually, ramp. You can program just one setting at a time or all three together.

As with a stationary cycle, resistance on an elliptical trainer determines how much effort it will take for you to keep your feet moving. Ramp levels describe how high or low you've set the angle of the ellipse. For instance, a high ramp mimics hiking, while a low ramp mimics cross-country skiing. The rate at which you move your legs determines the speed. The resistance will, of course, affect the speed at which you *can* move, but how you respond to the resistance is under your control. You could, for example, choose a low resistance and move quickly, or you could put the resistance up high and not be able to move smoothly. Ideally, says Florez, you want to be able to move at a comfortable, moderate speed, interspersed with occasional bursts of high intensity as well as high speeds.

High-quality elliptical trainers are expensive and may cost up to six times as much as a treadmill or a stationary bike, putting them out of range for many home exercisers. So most likely you'll use a trainer at a gym or fitness center, at least at first. If you fall in love with elliptical training and want to buy a machine for your home, here are some buying tips from experts.

Go for range. Look for a variety of ramp settings and intensity levels in an elliptical machine. If the ellipse itself isn't expansive and doesn't offer ramp and intensity changes, then the workout isn't nearly as effective.

The Precor EFX models, for example, use an oval-shaped collection of gears, pedals, and flywheels that allow

A Workout with Options Galore

To give your lower body a total workout on an elliptical trainer, mix and match the settings to mimic a number of sports. Each leg motion works different muscles in different ways, says J. Zack Barksdale, an exercise physiologist at the Cooper Aerobics Center in Dallas.

Cross-country skiing motion. Set the ramp level on low. This exercise emphasizes the butt and hamstring muscles. Unless you're practicing for a skiing race, try to keep the pace and resistance level moderate so that you can move smoothly.

Hiking motion. Keep the ramp setting on high and increase the intensity on the machine, which will simulate climbing.

Jogging motion. If you keep the ramp setting at middle height, you'll be moving in a motion close to running. Although the movement will be similar, you won't have the strain of impact to contend with.

Put it all together. With so many options, you could move from sport to sport within one workout, or you could simply do a different "sport" each time you get on the equipment. Either way, your lower body reaps an amazing array of workout benefits.

the legs to move in their full range of motion, giving you a good workout. At retail, they sell for approximately $2,000 to $2,700. If you try less expensive machines, with less of an elliptical shape, you may find that you don't get the same range of motion, says Florez.

If you can afford it, consider a model with a control panel that offers various preprogrammed courses and that records how many calories you've burned.

Skip the handles. Some machines come with handles that allow you to move your arms back and forth—with resistance—while you're on the elliptical machine. "That doesn't increase calorie burning very much," says Florez. "To burn more calories, it's much more effective to buy a machine without handles and work your legs at a higher intensity without leaning on your arms."

Try various settings. As with a treadmill or a stationary bike, you'll want to get a sense of how the machine feels at different settings. Try different combinations of ramp and speed settings. Also, vary the resistance, which enables you to work at different levels of intensity. The higher the resistance, the more power you'll need to exert to get your feet moving.

Measure twice, buy once. Elliptical trainers are long— up to 5 feet long—and over 4 feet tall at their highest point. Measure the machine you're going to buy and the space in which you plan to use it. And make sure you have enough headroom when you're standing on the machine.

Don comfortable clothes. Elliptical trainers don't require a special outfit. As with most workouts, your best bet is a layer or two of loose-fitting, comfortable clothing made of fabrics that wick away sweat. That way, you can peel off a layer as you work up a sweat. After a few workouts, you'll find what works best for you, says Florez.

Getting Started

When you first step onto an elliptical trainer, you'll probably start going backward. "This just tends to be the natural movement," says Florez. That's fine for a minute or two, but studies (and personal trainers) have found that going backward doesn't work the legs as effectively as forward motion. You will burn slightly more calories by going in reverse, says J. Zack Barksdale, an exercise physiologist at the Cooper Aerobics Center in Dallas, but not enough to make up for the potential strain you're putting on your knees.

Instead, simply place your feet on the footpads and push forward slightly. The trainer will begin to move your legs in the elliptical shape; all you have to do is follow along. The higher the level of resistance, the harder you'll have to push.

Go slowly. While you may be tempted to power your way through the virtual hills and valleys over which the elliptical machine can take you, stay in the midrange of the ellipse at first, advises Barksdale, who has put numerous people on elliptical training programs. "The wide range of motion the ellipse machine can take you through is great, but you need to work up to it."

Furthermore, people with lower-back problems may find this kind of exercise jarring, so consult your physician before working out on an elliptical trainer, Barksdale notes.

Keep your hands free. Getting your balance on an elliptical machine can be a little tricky at first. But bear in mind that you'll burn far more calories if you let go of the handles than if you hang on, says Barksdale. Allow your arms to swing freely, or try a little of a pumping action, he advises.

Keep your head straight. It may be easy to get distracted and look around or talk to someone while you're on the trainer, but twisting your torso is a no-no. To keep your knees in line with your feet and avoid injury, always point your head straight ahead, warns Barksdale.

Hiking

Breathe deeply. Smell the clean air, the flowers, the pine trees. Look around. See the blue sky, the green leaves, the white daisies, the yellow buttercups. Listen. It's quiet. Even the birds and crickets sound peaceful and serene. Stop. Take a drink from your water bottle and feel how cool the water is against your throat. Walk and feel the crunch of leaves underneath your feet, the craggy bark of the maples and oaks against your fingers, the crisp air drifting over your face. Oh, look! A doe and her fawn.

"Hiking is like walking, with one major difference: It takes you to new and exciting terrain," says Dan Heil, Ph.D., assistant professor of exercise physiology at Montana State University in Bozeman. So if you have been walking or running and hanker for variety, take to the trails.

Body-Shaping Benefits

Physiologically, hiking is walking turned up a notch or two. Here's how you can benefit.

- You'll burn more calories by hiking than by walking since climbing hills or walking on uneven terrain takes more energy.
- When you carry a pack of some kind (which most people do), the extra pounds further pump up your calorie burning.
- You'll give your quadriceps, hamstrings, gluteus maximus, and gluteus minimus (the major muscles in your hips, thighs, and buttocks) a good workout since hill walking forces your leg and thigh muscles to work even harder and more intensely than walking on flat terrain.
- If you use hiking poles, you'll tone your arm and back muscles, too.

The Right Footwear

You don't have to hoist a heavy overnight pack and sleep in a tent to hike. But you do need more than ordinary sneakers. You can get by with running or walking shoes, especially for short hikes on relatively flat terrain. But your feet will be a lot happier in hiking boots, especially if you have problems with weak ankles or balance.

Look for boots or trail shoes with lugged rubber soles. "You need a shoe with traction for going over rocks, dirt, leaves, and tree roots—all of which are slippery, especially when wet," says Dr. Heil. "And you need ankle support for stability." Whatever you do, don't wear loafers.

What Else You'll Need

Like fitness walking, hiking calls for a few other essentials.

Proper clothing. Thinking blue jeans? Think again. "Jeans are 100 percent cotton, which holds moisture against the skin if it gets wet from inside or outside the body," says Dr. Heil. "Instead, wear nylon shorts or hiking pants, and pullovers made from fabrics such as polypropylene or CoolMax, which keep moisture away from your body and dry quickly. In extremely cold weather, wear three layers. Use fabrics such as CoolMax, polypropylene, or ThermaStat blends as an inner layer to wick moisture away from the skin. For a middle layer, insulate by trapping a layer of warm air next to your body with fleece, wool, or BiPolar fabric. The outer layer should shield you from weather extremes. Wind jackets and pants of either Gore-Tex or Gore-Tex and fleece are all good outer protectors." If the weather is clear and only mildly cold, an inner and middle layer will suffice, adds Dr. Heil. You can find these clothes in sporting goods stores.

"If it's cool enough to wear a jacket, then you also need gloves and a hat since the largest source of heat loss is through the head and extremities," says Dr. Heil.

An extra pair of socks. If you're going on a long hike—more than half a day or so—wear two pairs of socks. The first (closest to your feet) should be made of a lightweight material that wicks away moisture, such as CoolMax. The outer layer should be made of a thicker material that protects your feet from rubbing against your shoe, like wool. "Switch to a new pair of both layers of socks about midway through the trip," says Dr. Heil. "It really feels better and is good for your skin."

Food. Okay, if you're just going for a 15-minute loop through the park, you will probably survive without something to eat. But if you're heading out for a couple of hours or longer, count on getting hungry. "You want snacks that are high in complex carbohydrates, such as granola bars, bananas, or a sandwich," says Dr. Heil.

Water. Anytime you exercise for an hour or more, you need to drink water to avoid even mild dehydration. So always carry bottled water or a water purifier. "Never drink water from a stream or creek because you don't know what might be upstream," says Dr. Heil. "Waste from livestock or wildlife may be just a few hundred yards away, or decomposing animals could be nearby, and you don't want to drink water that's passing over those areas before it makes its way down to you."

A walking stick. You can buy one, or you can simply use a sturdy stick you find on your trail (unless you're hiking in the desert). "Walking sticks are great if you have a back problem, bad knees, or trouble with balance," says Dr. Heil. "It's a third point on the ground. In fact, experienced hikers prefer two poles, which turn them into four-legged creatures." And they come in handy when crossing small streams.

One avid pole user is Diane Benedict, manager and trip leader for Mountain Fit, an organization in Bozeman that plans hiking adventures. "When descending, I find poles helpful to lessen the impact on my knees," she says. "And using one or two poles turns hiking into a great upper- and lower-body workout."

A map. Unless you can actually see the entire area that you're walking *while* you're walking, you need a map. "Call hiking clubs, walking clubs, a visitors' bureau, or a park headquarters where you plan to hike," suggests Dr. Heil.

Getting Started

You'll enjoy hiking more—and you'll be less likely to feel sore the next day—if you prepare ahead of time, says Benedict. Her suggestions are as follows.

Practice on stairs. The one type of walk you can't practice for in a gym is going downhill. "Coming down is what usually bothers people the first time they're out on a long hike, so climb down stadium stairs or just use the stairs in your office to get your quadriceps and knees ready for the descents," says Benedict.

Practice with your pack. Sure, your pocketbook weighs a ton, but how often do you sling it behind you and carry it up hills for 7 or 8 hours? If you're preparing for a long hike, load up your pack when you're going short distances. This way, you'll find out just how much weight you're comfortable with, and you'll also get to know the ins and outs of your pack.

Practice with your poles, too—it takes time to get used to using them before you can build up speed.

Adjust your stride. When you walk on flat terrain, you tend to take long strides. "But hiking requires small steps to remain steady on uneven ground," says Benedict.

Inline Skating

Want to exercise without feeling like it's exercise? Try inline skating. Far from the rickety ride you may remember from your childhood roller skates, inline skating is so smooth you almost feel like you're flying, says Kalinda Mathis, executive director of the International Inline Skating Association (IISA) in Wilmington, North Carolina, and an enthusiastic skater herself.

Further, if you're looking for a way to burn major calories while trimming your thighs, inline skating is made-to-order.

"Inline skating will give you legs to die for," says Carolyn Bradley of Wayne, Pennsylvania, who is an examiner for the International Inline Skating Association instructor certification program. "It's one of the best workouts you can get."

Body-Shaping Benefits

If you're game, here's what you can expect from inline skating.

- You'll tone and strengthen your lower body and torso, including your calves, thighs, buttocks, and, to a lesser degree, your tummy.
- You'll get a cardiovascular workout roughly comparable to running, without stressing your joints as much.
- You'll burn about as much fat and calories as treadmill running, stepping, or rowing but have a lot more fun along the way.

Psychological Benefits

Simply put, inline skating feels a lot more like playing than working. And that's no small perk in a world where grown-ups have few opportunities to let loose and have wind-in-your-face, fast, and giggly fun.

"You're outside, not in the gym. You're moving fast. The word a lot of people use to describe the feeling is freedom," says Mathis.

You can skate by yourself, focusing on your thoughts, or with a crowd. You can even do it with your kids, solving the problem of when to exercise for busy mothers.

Whether you prefer to go solo or social, inline skating is a stress-relieving activity, according to Mathis.

The Right Footwear

Inline skates are nothing like the metal contraptions you clamped to your play shoes with a skate key when you were in grade school. Basically, an inline skate is more like a sturdy ice skate with a series of wheels, bearings, and a brake built into a double-shelled boot with a buckle and lacing.

The number-one criterion in choosing a skate is comfort, says Mathis. Since skate prices start at about $100 and a high-quality pair of skates will cost between $150 and $300, it makes sense to rent several styles and brands before you commit. Some local sports equipment shops rent them out by the day.

Women's skates for women's feet. Most women prefer skates designed for women's feet, notes Mathis. They're built on a narrower last (the mold used for making footwear) than men's skates.

Start with a recreational skate. Compared with recreational skates, fitness skates are lighter, have a lower-cut boot, and larger wheels (76 to 80 versus 72 to 76 millimeters). As a beginner, you'll probably want to start on a recreational skate; later, should you commit to power workouts on wide, smooth surfaces, you may want to switch to a more high-performance fitness skate.

What Else You'll Need

When you walk or run, you're generally traveling at a speed of 3 to 8 miles per hour—a pretty leisurely clip. Inline skaters travel on hard surfaces at much faster speeds—anywhere from 10 to 25 miles per hour. Pebbles, deep sidewalk cracks, or other objects can trip up your wheels. Sooner or later, you'll fall. Unless you wear protective gear, you can fracture your wrist, arm, or collarbone, cautions Richard A. Schieber, M.D., of the National Center for Injury Prevention and Control in Atlanta. Here's what you'll need.

Wrist guards. When you fall, you tend to fall forward, putting your hand out to break your fall. Padded plastic wrist guards dissipate the impact—you slide along the ground on impact, saving your wrist from a sprain or a fracture from the impact. "Wrist guards are absolutely necessary," says Dr. Schieber.

Knee and elbow pads. Injuries to the knees and elbows are less common than injuries to the wrists, but you still want to protect your lower body from scrapes and bumps. Protective pads help cushion your fall so you don't leave part of your skin behind.

A helmet. Since a collision with the pavement or a vehicle can be catastrophic, you want to protect your brain. A biking helmet is better than an inline skating helmet because it must meet certain standards. All bicycle helmets made or sold in the United States have to meet federal safety standards set by the Consumer Product Safety Commission (CPSC). Dr. Schieber recommends a CPSC-certified bicycle helmet, but he says any helmet is better than none.

Clothing. What you wear to skate should accommodate your pads (jeans may not be comfortable with knee pads) and otherwise be comfortable and nonrestrictive. Most skaters choose exercise shorts on warm days or leggings on chilly days, plus comfortable tops that allow them to freely pump their arms.

Getting Started

Inline skating may look easy, but don't let that fool you into thinking you can just strap on a pair of skates and hit the sidewalk. Watching the neighborhood kids whiz by, you may think it certainly doesn't seem like a dangerous sport. But if you don't know what you're doing—and don't know how to stop or brace yourself for a fall—you could get hurt.

"Learning some basic moves and wearing the right equipment can greatly minimize your chances of hurting yourself," says Craig Young, M.D., medical director of sports medicine at the Medical College of Wisconsin in Milwaukee.

First, learn how to brake. In a study of more than 300 recreational inline skaters by doctors at the department of orthopedic surgery at the Medical College of Wisconsin in Milwaukee, nearly 15 percent stopped by skating off into the grass. Another 3 percent stopped by voluntarily falling. Neither method is much fun.

Proper braking on inline skates isn't difficult, says Mathis, but it doesn't come as second nature to newcomers. Save yourself time—and potential bruises: Call a sporting goods store that sells inline skates, or your local parks and recreation department, and sign up for an individual or group lesson so an instructor can show you how to glide, stride, and, most important, stop.

Dr. Schieber agrees. He strongly urges taking lessons from an instructor (as opposed to a friend). "When inline skating, you go fast from the first stroke," he notes. "You might not have the needed balance and agility from the start, and you need to learn how to fall. Remember, the skate is attached to your foot. You can't just 'jump off' at the first sign of trouble." Contact IISA at 201 North Front Street, Suite 306, Wilmington, NC 28401, for a list of instructors if you can't find one on your own.

Find a smooth, safe place to get started. Bradley, a former figure skater, recommends an empty parking lot, maybe early on a weekend morning, or an uncrowded bike path. "Definitely don't start skating on the street," she says.

The ideal place for any inline skating is a roller rink, adds Dr. Schieber.

Relax. Bend your knees and keep your hands in front of you as you glide your feet slowly and smoothly in front of each other, says Mathis. The rhythm will soon come easily to you.

Skate often. Inline skating may feel a little awkward at first, acknowledges Mathis. Commit to skating in short but regular sessions. "Practice really does make perfect in inline skating. The body starts to memorize where it should be over your skates to be comfortable," she says.

Jogging

Jogging gives you more bang for your buck than walking since it uses the same muscle groups but burns calories faster, says Ellen Glickman-Weiss, Ph.D., associate professor of exercise physiology in the department of exercise, leisure, and sports at Kent State University in Ohio.

"You can generally figure on burning 100 calories a mile," says Dr. Glickman-Weiss. "Walking 1 mile may take you 15 to 20 minutes; jogging will take you half as long. Both are tremendous for overall fitness benefits," she explains. Simply defined as running slowed down, jogging offers less risk of injury than full-out running, while it provides top-notch aerobic benefits.

Body-Shaping Benefits

Whether you jog on a treadmill or through a dew-sprinkled park, slow running provides a wealth of physical payoffs.

- You work both the large and the small muscle groups of your calves, thighs, buttocks, and hips and, in a less pronounced way, your waist and abdominal muscles.

- You use up fat stores, big time. And you'll burn about 102 calories per mile if you weigh 150 pounds.
- You'll raise your metabolic rate even after your running shoes are back in the closet. According to researchers at the University of Colorado, the resting metabolic rates of middle-aged women runners stayed steady as they grew older, while sedentary women gained weight and body fat as their resting metabolisms slowed. In the long run, older runners burn up to 600 additional calories a week (equal to 9 pounds a year!). "That doesn't even count the calories burned when they run," notes Pamela P. Jones, research assistant professor of kinesiology and applied physiology at the University of Colorado at Boulder.

The Right Footwear

Fortunately for joggers, manufacturers have come a long way in designing shoes to accommodate the sizes and running styles of virtually any woman, at prices that generally range from $50 to $100. Here's what to look for, according to Dr. Glickman-Weiss.

Shoes for *your* feet. Reading running shoe reviews can help you decide which of the dozens of shoe makes and models might best meet your needs, says Dr. Glickman-Weiss. Also consult knowledgeable salesclerks at sporting goods stores or athletic shoe stores. Take your old shoes along. Worn spots show whether you run more on the outside or the inside of your foot and which areas need the most support.

Enough wiggle room. A wide toe box is vital to give the front of your foot enough room when the force of your foot is pushed forward. Women with wide feet may want to check out running shoes designed specifically for women, from companies such as Ryka, which

Make Jogging More Fun

Here's how, says Ellen Glickman-Weiss, Ph.D., associate professor of exercise physiology in the department of exercise, leisure, and sports at Kent State University in Ohio.

Say okay to a fund-raising 5-K. The competition, free T-shirt, and opportunity to help raise money for worthy causes can motivate you to stick with your program.

Increase distance, not speed. In one study of women who ran recreationally, those who ran the most miles per week had the narrowest waists and hips, regardless of how fast they ran.

Don't run every day. Running too often increases the risk of knee, hip, and tendon problems and of other common injuries. Three to five days a week is fine. Beginners shouldn't run more than 15 miles a week. At that point the stresses on your body outweigh the benefits.

Increase your weekly distance by no more than 10 percent a week. If you're jogging 3 days a week for 30 minutes a day, for example, and covering 3 miles, increase by no more than 1 mile total the first week.

Stick to flat, smooth surfaces. Minimize impact by sticking to a soft, smooth, unbanked cinder track or an artificial surface. The same goes for soft, smooth dirt trails. Avoid asphalt and concrete.

Alternate jogging with other activities. Swimming, water aerobics, cycling, stairclimbing, rowing, and cross-country skiing give your feet and legs a respite from the constant pounding of running, while they work other muscle groups.

makes shoes exclusively for women, New Balance, and Saucony.

All-weather, all-surface tread and materials. If you're going to be running in rain and snow, look for a shoe made from weather-tight fabric, with a hard-core outer tread. If you're a treadmill runner, this isn't important.

Replacements, as needed. Buy a new pair of shoes every 6 months or 600 miles. At that point shoes start to fall apart, even if they still look good. You can prolong the life of your running shoes by wearing them only to run.

Treadmill Tips

If you find that rain, sleet, and snow keep you from jogging, try treadmill running at a gym. If you find yourself sticking to it (and you can afford it), consider a treadmill for your home. To save money, shop at a secondhand sports equipment store.

Choose a body-friendly model. Some treadmills have a built-in suspension, like shock absorbers on a car, to minimize the impact on weak hips or knees, says Edmund Burke, Ph.D., professor of exercise science at the University of Colorado in Colorado Springs and author of the *Complete Home Fitness Handbook*.

These machines approximate the impact of running on a soft surface, says Dr. Glickman-Weiss. They're also sturdier and better able to accommodate heavier walkers and runners than lightweight units that you can stow under a bed, she adds.

Go for a test jog. If you decide to buy, go dressed for action to a reputable fitness showroom. Run on many treadmills, looking for a shock-absorbing platform, plus a belt wide and long enough for your comfort, and handrails you like.

Know you can stop. So that you can stop without risking an injury, make sure the treadmill has a device that will immediately stop the belt in case you run into trouble, advises Dr. Burke.

Getting Started

Unless you're already in shape, work up to jogging gradually. Start out walking, then increase the distance and then the intensity of your walks.

Jog at a slow pace for 10, then 15, then 20 minutes, making sure you're not so out of breath that you can't talk to a partner while running, says Dr. Glickman-Weiss. When you're ready for more, run longer, not faster.

Jumping Rope

For the busy woman on a budget, jumping rope is the ultimate calorie-burning exercise. It doesn't take a lot of time, it's inexpensive, and it's high-intensity.

Body-Shaping Benefits

Women who want to lose weight are ideal candidates for jumping rope, says Ken Solis, M.D., an emergency room physician at Beaver Dam Community Hospital in Greenfield, Wisconsin, and the author of Ropics, a book of exercises he developed for the jump rope. Among the rewards:

- You'll burn calories—110 to 130 per 10 minutes if you weigh 150 pounds. Jumping rope is on a par with running when it comes to calorie burn.
- You'll improve endurance, coordination, balance, and timing.
- You'll strengthen your bones as well as your muscles; this is a great bonus because it helps prevent osteoporosis.

The Right Footwear

Since you're going to be doing a lot of bouncing on the balls of your feet, wearing the right shoes is important. Otherwise, you could sprain an ankle or tear a tendon. You'll need a high-quality pair of aerobic or cross-training shoes to give you cushioning and support in all the right places, says exercise physiologist Carla Sottovia, assistant fitness director at the Fitness Cooper Center in Dallas. When you're in the store, cast your inhibitions to the wind and jump up and down to make sure the shoes fit right. As for those old tennis shoes, running shoes, or sneakers in your closet—use them for other sports, she says.

What Else You'll Need

Once upon a time, an old clothesline might have served as a jump rope. Now you have many more choices—and it's also important to choose the right bra and mat. Here are the possibilities.

Spring for the swivel. The rope should swivel within the handles or at the handles so that the rope doesn't twist on itself while you're jumping, says Dr. Solis.

Choose right. Jump ropes are made of many materials. Starting out, you might choose a segmented rope (otherwise known as a beaded rope) or a rope made of woven cotton or synthetic material. A segmented, or beaded, rope has a nylon cord at the center that's strung with cylindrical plastic beads that look like hollow noodles. A woven rope—made of nylon, cotton, or polypropylene—resembles the old-fashioned kind of jump rope, and it won't sting as much if you happen to swat your back, Dr. Solis notes from personal experience.

After you've advanced a bit, you might choose a speed rope or a licorice rope. They're made from vinyl plastic, and they're light and fast. Leather ropes are just as fast as speed ropes, but they wear out sooner. Some advanced jump ropers who are in very good physical condition choose weighted ropes, which can weigh up to 6 pounds. Needless to say, you don't want a weighted rope until you're very confident about your swinging and timing, says Dr. Solis.

Jump for Joy!

Keep these guidelines in mind as jumping becomes a regular part of your life, says Ken Solis, M.D., an emergency room physician in Greenfield, Wisconsin, and author of *Ropics*, a book of exercises he developed for the jump rope.

Warm to the task. Start with an easy, two-footed jump for a few minutes until your muscles get warmed up. After you feel comfortable, try a light jog step.

Alternate between high- and low-impact jumping. When you stop to take a breather, try marching in place for a while.

Mix and match. For a high-intensity interval workout, combine jumping rope with circuit training. For instance, after a warmup, alternate jumping with pushups, triceps dips, and squats.

Be very varied. There are many variations on jumping rope, such as the heel-dig jump: With each jump, you bring one leg in front of your body as if you were digging in your heel. It looks like a variation on a Cossack dance.

Join others. Skipping rope with other people helps you beat boredom and stick with your routine. Many classes are held in conjunction with kickboxing or martial arts classes, and they're offered at aerobics studios. Local gyms, YWCAs, kickboxing schools, and martial arts schools are likely to have information.

Measure for leisure. When a rope is the right length, you can hold it at waist level and hardly move your hands, and it will clear your head and feet with no problem. (If you have to circle your arms around, the rope's too short; if it bounces and hits your ankles, it's too long.) To get a comfortable length, stand with one or both feet in the middle of the rope, then lift the handles as high as they'll go. If they reach your armpits, you have what you want, says Dr. Solis. Some ropes are adjustable, and others can be shortened just by putting in a couple of overhand knots near the handles.

Cradle your top. You probably know by now whether or not you're more comfortable in an exercise bra—but this is a sport where you might even want two. Women who take a bra size 36 or larger usually do best by layering two running bras on top of each other and then wearing a close-fitting T-shirt or tank on top of that, says Sottovia.

Find the space. "Even though it's convenient to skip rope at home, it's sometimes hard to find enough room above you and around you," says Dr. Solis. If you're average height, you'll need at least a 9-foot ceiling, with plenty of space around you. The lawn won't work, because the rope gets tangled in the grass, and carpet slows you down. So you might head for the basement, garage, or patio. That's fine, as long as you're on a surface that has a little give to it, like wood or hard rubber, says Dr. Solis. You don't want to jump on hard concrete or tile, he warns. Those surfaces don't give you any bounce, and they're murder on your joints.

Go to the mat. You can convert a thick carpet to a jump-friendly surface by using a plastic mat that is usually sold to be placed under an office desk or chair, says Dr. Solis. These are available at larger office supply stores.

To convert the floor in a garage or a spare room into a jump-friendly surface, invest in plastic interlocking tiles, says Budd Pickett, executive director of the United States Amateur Jump Rope Federation (USAJRF). These are not soft mats but flooring used in indoor courts for sports such as volleyball, gymnastics, and jumping rope, he explains. To locate a store near you that sells interlocking tiles, write to Sport Court at 939 South 700 West, Salt Lake City, UT 84104.

A hard rubber mat or flooring, too, is good, according to Dr. Solis. Avoid squishy aerobics mats because they have too much give, he adds.

Getting Started

"If you're just starting out and haven't skipped rope in years, don't set out to jump for a certain amount of time," says Dr. Solis. Instead, ease into it.

Skip the skip. Begin jumping with both feet, but try to do it without that little skip between jumps. Jump just high enough to clear the rope and bring it over fast so you don't have time for that extra hop. Start out at the easiest pace you can without having to add the hop.

Pedal your feet. For variation, try jogging from foot to foot as you jump. The motion is more like pedaling a bike or light jogging than jumping up and down. You control the intensity by how fast you "jog" through your rope.

Keep your elbows in and wrists relaxed. With your elbows tucked close by your sides, your arms should barely move while you're skipping rope. Swing the rope with a relaxed motion of your forearms and wrists.

Stick to the low jump. "There's no need to lift more than 1 inch off the ground," says Sottovia. You should rise just high enough so that the rope can clear the space between your feet and the mat.

Stop when you want to. If you're tired after a minute or two of jumping, just take a break—then try again when you feel like it.

Power Walking

If you're like a lot of women who walk to lose weight and get in shape, you've probably been walking around your neighborhood religiously for months. You know every kid, every cat, and every dog within 2 miles of your house. You're out there, rain or shine. There's just one problem: You're getting a little bored. You don't want to jog, but you would like to somehow take your walks to the next level—burn a few more calories or get slimmer sooner.

Power walking is the sport for you. While the average walker usually covers about 3 miles in an hour-long walk, a power walker strives to do at least 4 miles in the same time period. Serious power walkers can eventually do about 6 miles in an hour, but that's going pretty darn fast. In fact, it's faster than some people run.

Most women will simply strive to bump up their 20-minute-per-mile stroll to a 15-minute-mile power hike. Power walking is any walking done as exercise, rather than just recreation, according to Jeff Salvage, a Medford, New Jersey, junior national coordinator of U.S. Track and Field, a governing body of the U.S. Track Team.

"Power walking is the obvious next step for women who've made walking a habit," says Salvage, who is also a racewalking coach and author of *Walk like an Athlete*.

Body-Shaping Benefits

Here's what you can expect when you power walk regularly.

- If you are a regular walker but find that you have to walk long periods of time in order to burn as much fat as you want, power walking will help you burn calories in less time.
- You can burn 198 to 250 calories per mile if you weigh 150 pounds.
- You will tone all the muscles in your lower body, including the gluteus maximus (the large muscle in your buttocks), the hamstrings (along the backs of your thighs), and the quadriceps (in the fronts of your thighs).

The Right Footwear

"Try on as many walking shoes as possible before you buy a pair," says Carol Espel, a Walk Reebok master trainer and the executive fitness director of Equinox Fitness Clubs of New York. "You want to look for shoes that are lightweight and that breathe. (Look for mesh on the top or sides of the shoe.) The forefoot of the shoe should be flexible, so it bends fairly easily," she says.

"A slanted, or beveled, heel makes it easier to walk with a heel-to-toe motion, which is one of the techniques of power walking. It puts less strain on your shin muscles, thus avoiding shin splints," adds Espel. "Ultimately, though, you have to find the shoe that's most comfortable for you."

What Else You'll Need

While walking is the easiest form of exercise, power walking requires some technique. "It's not just a matter of walking faster," says Espel.

"The difference between a 17-minute-per-mile 'health walker' and a 13-minute-per-mile 'power walker' is technique," notes Salvage, who coaches women of all levels and ages.

Here's what you'll need for your metamorphosis.

A trail or a treadmill. While there's nothing wrong with simply walking around your neighborhood, if you want to power walk, you'll want to know exactly how long your training ground is. To do that, you can map out a course that's 4 to 5 miles long, do laps on a high school track, or walk on a treadmill that automatically records your pace and distance. Each of these choices has its own benefits.

"Getting started can be as easy as walking through a park or your neighborhood, which is wonderful because of the scenery and varying terrain," says Espel. "Tracks are good because you can concentrate on technique and don't have to worry about traffic."

Breathing in the fresh air and letting the wind pass over your body is healthy, says Salvage. Treadmills, on the other hand, allow you to pinpoint your pace and distance, which is also very helpful in the beginning.

Start with a warmup, advises Espel. Walk at a comfortable pace for about 5 minutes or until you break out in a light sweat. Then stretch your quadriceps, hips, hamstrings, and shins.

Water. If you're accustomed to waiting until you get home from your stroll to rehydrate, it's time to change. "You must carry a water bottle with you," says Espel. "Your power walks will be more intense than your old walks, so it's important to have water before, during, and after your workout." Drink at least a cup of water before starting out, a cup or more while you're walking, and still more water afterward, she recommends.

If you don't want to carry the water in your hand, invest in a fanny pack or waist pack that's big enough to hold a bottle of water. Or buy one that has a strap in which to place the bottle. It's a must.

A progress log. Morphing from a walker to a power walker means keeping track of your progress. "Your log doesn't have to be fancy or formal," says Espel. "Just write down when you walked, how far you went, how it felt, and how long it took you."

Getting Started

To hone your power walking technique, you'll need to focus on your feet, your hips, and your arms. Espel offers these tips.

Feet: Think heel-toe. Take quick, short steps, not long, extended strides. "Your goal is to pick up your feet faster," says Espel. "To do that, you have to focus on rolling your foot from heel to toe. Come down on your heel, with your toes up, then roll through your foot, pushing off on your toes when that leg is behind you." It should almost feel as if you're rolling forward.

Hips: Think steady and straight. Lots of people, thinking power walkers look as if they're waddling, assume those walkers are rocking their hips from side to side. Not so. Instead, with power walking you use your hips as an extension of your legs, so each hip moves forward and back (but stays level) as its accompanying leg moves forward. You're not pushing your hips, says Espel, but you're utilizing their power.

Arms: Think propulsion. Your arms play a big role in how fast you walk. Keep them stationary and your stroll will never turn into a power walk. "The faster you pump your arms, the faster your body will move," says Espel. "That doesn't mean, though, that you want your arms to swing wildly without control." Instead, your arms should be bent at a 90-degree angle and move steadily forward and back, but your fists should never go back farther than your hips or go higher than your sternum.

Eyes: Look ahead. Use your eyes to aim for a landmark far ahead of you, Espel suggests. "You should be looking at the horizon or focused on a spot down the block. That focus will add to your momentum as well as ensure that your posture is correct."

Posture: Lean forward from the ankles. "Imagine yourself looking like a ski jumper in midair," says Espel. "That's almost the angle at which you want your body." In other words, there should be no bend in your waist.

Here are some equations.

- If you're just beginning to change your walk into a power walk, you might need music with 110 beats per minute, which is a 19-minute-per-mile pace—just a tad faster than the usual 3-mile-an-hour pace you might be accustomed to for exercise.
- If you're doing a solid power walk, pick music with 130 beats per minute, which translates to a 15-minute-per-mile pace.
- If you're going full throttle at the breakneck speed of a 13-minute-per-mile pace, pick music with 150 beats per minute.

Whole body: Stretch afterward. Power walking is harder on many lower-body parts than slow walking is, so you'll need to make sure that you stretch properly afterward, just as a professional athlete does after she works out or competes.

Specific areas to stretch? Again, the hips, quadriceps, hamstrings, and shins. "Shin pain is probably the number-one complaint of fitness walkers," says Espel. "Ideally, your shins should adjust to a walk within the first 5 minutes. If they hurt or ache, you're going too fast." She suggests you slow your pace or try walking backward—retro walking, it's called. This takes all the pressure off the shins. Once your shins feel better, resume walking forward.

Spinning

Also known as studio cycling, Spinning is basically road cycling brought indoors. It's done on a specially designed workout bike and is set to music or a series of visualizations.

Even if you tried stationary cycling and hated it, you'll love Spinning. For one thing, it simulates riding a bike more than stationary cycling does. A Spinning bike has a weighted wheel, called a flywheel, that picks up speed when you pedal, so you feel as if you're actually going down (or up) hills or just riding along a country road. You can also stand on a Spin bike in order to climb the "hills" with more power (and thus change the muscles you're working in your legs). Finally, Spinning is a group activity. A certified Spinning instructor leads your ride—sometimes using visualization, sometimes using speed work, and sometimes combining every move you can do, making for some of the most intense—and addictive—workouts most women have ever experienced, says Ron Crawford, a certified Spinning instructor from Niles, Ohio, and president of World of Fitness, which operates two fitness facilities.

Body-Shaping Benefits

Here's what you can expect when you spin regularly.

- You'll burn 600 to 800 calories an hour—about as much as rowing on a machine at race pace.
- You'll tone your entire lower body, especially your butt and the fronts of your thighs.
- If you do a lot of standing and sitting intervals (known as jumps), you'll strengthen your abdominal muscles.

Psychological Benefits

Spinning is a true mind–body experience. The instructor will choose from a variety of "rides," each of which will add to your mental pleasure in a specific way. For example, some Spinning instructors lead their students through imaginary trips through the south of France or down the coast of California. Others lead you through intervals that simulate a road race. And others simply have you close your eyes and stay in touch with the way your body feels as you pedal through a variety of intensities and positions.

"It's almost a Zen experience," says Deborah Gallagher, a certified personal trainer and certified Spinning instructor in Vacaville, California. "You're moving in a repetitive fashion along with the music, but you don't have to worry about coordination. When I look at my students, I see joy on their faces."

The Right Footwear

Like the pedals on traditional racing bikes, Spinning bike pedals consist of a "cage," which holds your sneakered foot steady, and a "lock" for bike shoes. "Locking your foot into the pedal helps you move your legs more smoothly," explains Crawford. "But not everyone likes the feel of bike shoes." Most bike pedal manufacturers have a universal lock, which means that most bike shoes will fit into any bike pedal, Spinning or otherwise.

What Else You'll Need

Very few people purchase their own Spinning bikes because so much of the sport's appeal is its group atmosphere. So chances are you'll join a class. If you do, here's what Gallagher suggests you bring along.

Water. Spinning bikes include built-in water bottle holders for a very good reason—you're going to need to stay hydrated during the class. Most of the holders will fit a small bottle of water—preferably one with a pop-up spout so you don't have to interrupt your ride to open up your bottle.

A towel. You'll need a small hand towel, not only to sop up the sweat from your forehead but also to wipe down your bike before someone else gets ready to use it.

Bike shorts (maybe). Like riding any bike, Spinning can irritate a tender tush (or other sensitive spots). "Bike shorts have extra padding in the butt to cushion you," says Gallagher. "They're available at most sporting goods stores."

A gel seat. Some gyms provide bike seats filled with gel, while others expect you to bring your own. "Available at sporting goods stores, gel seats have a lot more give than a traditional bike seat," notes Gallagher. "Some people prefer gel seats to bike shorts—especially if you don't look great in close-fitting shorts or can't find them in your size."

Getting Started

Yes, Spinning is a tough aerobic and lower-body workout. But as with all exercises, you have to start slowly and progress gradually.

Take a beginner class. "Most gyms offer a 'Begin to Spin' class for rookies," says Crawford. "The instructor will show you how to adjust your bike so that you're safe and comfortable as you ride." The bike needs to be adjusted for your height. If the seat is too low or the pedal tension is too high, for example, you may experience knee pain.

Begin to Spin classes are not as intense as intermediate or advanced Spinning workouts, and the instructors will explain directives used in class, such as "continue cadence" and "lighten up." They'll also check on your form, either as they spin or by walking around. Most gyms have mirrored walls, so you can check out your form as you go, too.

The five basic Spinning moves are:

Seated flat. This is the basic sitting position on the bike. You'll use this for warmup, cooldown, and speed work.

Seated hill. This is pretty much the same position as the seated flat, but when you increase the resistance of the flywheel, your butt will slide back a little bit in order to give your legs more power to pedal. Try to keep your upper body relaxed, and, most important, don't jam the pedals on the downstroke. Your leg motion should remain fluid even though you're working hard.

Standing hill. Once the resistance forces you to incorporate more leg power, you'll naturally want to stand up. Your pedaling will slow down, but your legs will work very hard and you'll feel the resistance of the bike. Not only will this burn lots of calories, but it will really work the muscles of your legs and butt.

Running. It's not really running, but your legs will be moving quickly. In a standing position, you'll decrease the resistance on the flywheel, move your legs and torso slightly ahead of the seat, and—with less resistance than you use when on a standing hill—push the pedals as quickly as possible, without losing control of the bike. Spinners usually "run" after a good warmup to increase their heart rates and get to the next level of exertion.

Jumping. This is not really jumping, but it is a very high intensity move. Keeping the bike at a fairly high and consistent resistance level, you'll do some interval work. Without changing your pedaling rhythm, or cadence, you'll stand up for a measured amount of time, then sit down for the same amount of time. You have to make sure that you're not throwing your weight forward or pushing your legs down hard; the motion should be smooth and fluid. Some instructors change the length of the intervals from four counts to another number.

Vary your hand positions. Since Spinning simulates actual road riding, your hand positions will also vary according to the ride, says Gallagher.

Close together, used when you're seated. Your hands are next to each other, not grasping the handlebars too tightly. Your elbows and shoulders are always relaxed, with your knuckles slightly higher than your wrists. Your elbows should flare out a little bit.

Wider apart, used for seated climbing and jumping. Your hands are slightly separated and relaxed. Don't hold the handlebars too tightly.

On the ends of the handlebars, used only for standing hill part of your workout, your hands are at the outermost edges of the handlebars, with your knuckles facing out and your fingers wrapped around the bar. "This is the position used when you're out riding your bike with others and you're trying to catch up with them," says Gallagher.

Aim for balance between speed (how fast you pedal) and resistance (how hard it is to pedal). You want to keep some resistance on the flywheel; otherwise, it will feel as if your legs are moving out of control.

Ride for yourself. Although Spinning is a group activity, there is absolutely no competition. "No one can tell at what resistance level you're riding," says Crawford. "And no one will force you to stand when everyone else is standing or to jump if everyone else is jumping." Tune in to the experience of how the ride feels for you, he says, not how you're doing in relation to anyone else in the class.

Step Aerobics

A form of exercise involving high-intensity, low-impact movement choreographed on and around an adjustable platform, step aerobics was born in the late 1980s. During a step aerobic workout, you'll step on, over, and around a bench, all in time to heart-pumping music. It's one of the few exercise fads that have become fitness staples.

You don't have to be highly coordinated to do step aerobics (although the more proficient you become, the easier the choreography is), says Gin Miller, the inventor of step aerobics, creator of Step Reebok, and star of Reebok Step Training videos, in Canton, Georgia. And you don't have to perform step aerobics at a gym. You can buy a step bench and various step videos in sporting goods stores and catalogs, which makes step aerobics one of the least expensive—and most effective—at-home workouts you can try.

Body-Shaping Benefits

Here's what you can expect when you do step aerobics regularly.

- You'll burn lots of fat since step aerobics is a high-intensity exercise.
- You'll tone and shape the muscles in your lower body, especially your butt, thighs, and calves.
- If you concentrate on keeping your abdominals contracted while you step, you'll tone and strengthen your abdominal muscles.
- You can burn about 300 calories per half-hour, using a 6-inch step, if you weigh 150 pounds.

Psychological Benefits

Like other aerobic exercise, step aerobics will improve your mood as well as your ability to think creatively.

"As a bonus, step aerobics can also help women who feel klutzy get over their fears of choreography or footwork," says Miller. "It doesn't require as much coordination as dancing, yet you're still exercising to music and using some low-impact dance moves."

The Right Footwear

You'll want support while you do your step aerobics routine, so a good pair of aerobic shoes is your best bet. Look for flexible shoes that have plenty of cushioning and arch support on the bottom, recommends Tamilee Webb, the choreographer of numerous step videos and author of The Step Up Fitness Workout, who lives in San Diego. Some women prefer higher-cut shoes that give their ankles extra support.

What Else You'll Need

Once you've laced up your shoes, you'll need a step bench—a low and wide platform with graduated risers so you can increase step height as you become more experienced at step aerobics. Some risers are attached to the step and simply fold under it when you want to change the step height.

Here's what to look for in a step bench, according to Webb.

Sturdy construction. Because you'll be stepping up and down on the bench, it should feel as solid as any step you would climb in your house. Likewise, any risers that come with the step should also be solid and not wobble at all as you go up and down the bench.

A step that is wide and long enough. You need plenty of room for both of your feet on the bench. Some choreography won't work with a narrow step, so if the step bench is too narrow, it's not a good buy. You should also be able to take at least one step out to the side while you're on the bench. The ideal step is 2 feet wide and 3 feet long. You can buy shorter (and cheaper) step benches, but the longer and wider the bench is, the more intense you'll be able to make your workouts.

Getting Started

Step aerobics is a high-intensity exercise, so you'll want to begin your workout routine slowly. Experts recommend videotapes specifically geared toward beginners (such as those offered by instructors such as Gin Miller, Tamilee Webb, and Kathy Smith, for example).

Once you select a tape, here's how to use it.

Take baby steps. The basic step pattern goes "up-up, down-down": up with the right foot, up with the left foot, down with the right foot, down with the left foot. "It's just like the way a child first learns to climb a staircase," says Webb. "The most important thing to remember is that you have to place your whole foot on the step, not just your toes and not just the ball of your foot."

At first, you'll have to look to make sure your foot is in proper position. Eventually, you'll get a feel for where you're stepping, and you can look ahead, not down, and follow the tape or instructor.

Basic Step Is Just the Beginning

Once you become comfortable using beginner tapes at home, consider ratcheting up your routine. Noted step instructors Gin Miller and Tamilee Webb offer these suggestions.

Add some weight training. Some step instructors use both free weights and tubing after the step segment to work resistance training into their routines. These help you burn more calories and allow you to target the areas you want to tone the most, including your upper body.

Create your own workout. Use a combination of moves: *Low-intensity* moves include the basic step (up-up, down-down), knee lift (up-knee, down-down/up-knee, down-down), and over the top (where you travel over the step to the other side). *Moderate-intensity* moves are traveling movements (moving from side to side on the bench) and repeaters (standing with one foot on the bench and repeatedly bringing the other knee up). *High-intensity* moves may include lunges, leaps, hops, runs, and jumps. Make sure you perform airborne movements on the up accent only, cautions Miller.

Don't use music that's too fast. It shouldn't be as fast as traditional aerobic music. Look for songs with about 2 beats per second—120 beats per minute. But if you don't want to count beats, simply notice how you're feeling and moving during your workout. If you're tripping while you exercise, the music is simply too fast for stepping.

First, master the legs, then add your arms. When you're first learning to perform step aerobics, don't worry about moving your arms, even if the instructor on the workout tape is mixing her arms into the patterns. Instead, concentrate on getting the foot patterns down and feeling comfortable using the platform, says Miller. When you're ready, begin to incorporate the arm movements into your routine. Continuous arm movements increase your heart rate, and thus the number of calories you burn, by up to 10 percent.

Forget the hand weights. Hand weights can limit movement, and they can also cause pain and fatigue in your shoulders when used for long periods of time, cautions Webb.

Limit yourself to no more than four step workouts a week. Studies have shown that doing step aerobics more than four times a week markedly increases the chance of injury. So be happy that it's a high-intensity workout that will burn tons of calories in a very short amount of time.

Increase step height very gradually. The Reebok stepping platform—considered a "benchmark"-size step by experts—is 6 inches high. You can adjust the height by 2 inches at a time to make the advanced step bench a total height of up to 10 inches.

When you feel comfortable doing your step routine at the lowest height, add height 2 inches at a time, until your leg reaches a 60-degree angle or a comfortable step height. Only very tall or extremely advanced exercisers should use a step bench that's higher than 10 inches, says Miller. Step height (combined with your body weight) is the biggest variable in terms of how many calories you'll burn.

Stepping Machines

Are you intimidated by—yet envious of—those slender women moving up and down on the long line of stairclimbing machines at the gym? Well, there's a good reason these women are so svelte. Few workouts trim and tone your butt and thighs as efficiently as stepping.

"Like stairclimbing, using a step machine accomplishes two important jobs," says exercise physiologist Carla Sottovia, assistant fitness director at the Fitness Cooper Center in Dallas. It burns off overall fat, and it gives definition to the muscles of your lower body, including the gluteals (in your buttocks), hamstrings and quadriceps (in your thighs), and gastrocnemius (in your calves). As the excess fat melts away, the long, lean muscles underneath are revealed.

Although the terms *stepper* and *stairclimber* are used interchangeably, they are two different machines. Steppers work only your lower body. You balance on the handlebars, alternately pushing with one foot at a time. Climbers work the whole body.

"The key to being consistent with your stepping workouts is finding an effective form of distraction," says

Cedric X. Bryant, Ph.D., senior vice president of research and development/sports medicine at the StairMaster Corporation in Kirkland, Washington. "On a step machine, you can read, watch television, listen to music, or program the machine to vary your workouts. You can't very easily do that on stairs."

Body-Shaping Benefits

Repeatedly raising and lowering your body with either a stepper or a stairclimber uses all the large muscles in your hips, butt, thighs, and lower legs. As a result, stepping combines calorie burning (which uses fat as energy, so it comes off your body) with lower-body sculpting.

Here's what you can expect when you use a stepper regularly.

- You'll tone and strengthen your butt and thigh muscles, leaving you with a smaller butt and leaner thighs.
- You'll develop shapelier calf muscles.
- You'll burn 250 to 350 calories per half-hour if you weigh 150 pounds.

What You'll Need

Any type of athletic shoe or comfortable sneaker will work on a step machine, so you don't have to go out and buy elaborate footwear.

You'll find steppers or stairclimbers in most gyms, so you don't necessarily have to buy one—unless you want to. Like other forms of exercise equipment, such as treadmills and weight machines, step machines are convenient, but the good ones can run you some money.

Here are some questions to ask and features to think about when you're considering a step machine at a gym or shopping for a home model.

Is it sturdy? The equipment should be able to support your weight easily and remain steady even while you're in motion, says Sottovia. The more expensive machines are usually sturdier and a better buy for people who have a significant amount of weight to lose.

Is it the right size? Every step machine has a prescribed range of distance that the footpad can travel as you step. Some ranges are wider than others. It should be easy for you to stay in the midrange, or "sweet spot," of the step length. Likewise, the footpads should be big enough to hold your entire foot with room to spare. Try every machine to see which feels most comfortable to you, suggests Sottovia.

How does it work? There are two different kinds of step machine designs, dependent and independent. If you push down on one step of a dependent machine, the other step will rise, creating greater stress on the knee joint. Independent steps aren't connected by anything and involve more natural and less stressful movement, says Dr. Bryant.

Most brands of step machines offer display monitors with manual or programmed features that set and measure the time and intensity of your effort. The programs also help you check your progress and guide you through a variety of workouts. You don't need an elaborately programmed unit to get a good workout, though, says Dr. Bryant. Choose a machine based on how the equipment moves as you exercise, not the display features, he says.

What type of resistance does it use? Experts recommend buying hydraulic, cable, or chain steppers. Be careful, though, since hydraulic machines (which are less expensive) use oil, which can leak onto home carpeting.

Beat the Monotony of Endless Climbing

Supplement your workout with these suggestions.

Take the stairs—any stairs. Besides taking the steps and not the elevator at work, use the stairs for 10 minutes of exercise a few times a day, says exercise physiologist Carla Sottovia, assistant fitness director at the Fitness Cooper Center in Dallas. But don't wear dress pumps or heels. They throw you off balance and take a toll on your knees, especially when going down the stairs. Wear sneakers, or at least flats.

Get tough. The Stepmill is a tough but effective machine that looks like a flight of stairs and requires complete stairclimbing motion on 8-inch steps. The stairs keep revolving (like an escalator) so that you can climb them over and over again.

Add your upper body. To give your upper body a workout, look into a vertical climbing machine, such as the VersaClimber by Heart Rate. It's a lot like climbing a stationary ladder, and because you work your arms and legs in a full range of motion, you'll burn lots of calories.

Visualize a goal. Imagine you're climbing famous steps, like the Spanish Steps in Rome, Mayan ruins in Mexico, Telegraph Hill in San Francisco, or stairs to the top of the Statue of Liberty. Or set a long-range goal—like the equivalent of climbing Mount Everest. Find out how many steps it would take to reach your goal, then post it near your step machine or in your exercise log and chart your daily progress.

Leading brands of steppers include StairMaster, Tunturi, VersaClimber, and Tectrix.

Getting Started

Stepping might look as easy as marching, but stepping improperly can cost you 75 calories per workout. Bad form can also contribute to aches and pains during and after your workout. After all, you're not just bounding up the steps to answer the phone—you're stepping nonstop for half an hour. To step safely and effectively, you have to do it right. Here's how.

Warm up. As with any exercise, a good rule for stepping is "start slow, stop gradually," says Sottovia. "Warm up for 5 minutes with smaller steps on a low resistance level, then move into your workout with longer steps at a higher resistance. Slow down again at the end, and make sure you stretch your leg muscles afterward."

Don't lean on the rails. "When people lean, they tend to do about 20 to 25 percent less work than the machine credits them for because they aren't using their full body weight when they step," says Dr. Bryant. "If you're working so hard that you have to lean on the machine, lower the stepping speed. Your hands should rest lightly, if at all, on the handlebars."

Slow down. Stepping quickly doesn't mean you'll burn more calories. It's the force of your leg working against the step, not how fast you step, that determines the value of the workout. Your steps should cover the middle range of the whole length of the step, and your speed should be steady, not fast or choppy, according to Dr. Bryant.

Swimming

Few activities are as sensual and relaxing as swimming. And swimming may be the perfect way for a woman who needs to lose a few pounds to begin an exercise program because extra fat helps keep you buoyant, making it easier to swim better and faster. If you have a lot of weight to lose—50 pounds or more—swimming is a good way to get started.

"Swimming isn't weight-bearing—it doesn't subject your joints and bones to a lot of added impact," says Jane Katz, Ed.D., professor of health and physical education at the John Jay College of Criminal Justice of City University of New York and author of *The All-American Aquatic Handbook* and *Swimming for Total Fitness*. "You're expending a lot of energy, which burns calories, but you don't have to support the weight of your whole body while you do it."

If you start to swim and stick with it, you could wind up as sleek, slender, and elegant as a mermaid.

Body-Shaping Benefits

Here's what you can expect when you swim regularly.

- You'll burn as many calories as running, without stressing your knees or bones.
- You'll tone your abdomen and hips.
- You'll tone and strengthen your legs. As a bonus, you'll also firm up your chest and upper arms.

Psychological Benefits

Despite the anxiety many women feel about getting into a bathing suit, most women feel light and beautiful once they're actually in the water.

"In the water, your body feels as though it weighs one-tenth your actual weight," says Dr. Katz. "So many women feel graceful, sensuous, and feminine when they swim."

If you're substantially overweight, having the weight of your body off your bones and joints for an hour or so may also be a physical relief. "Many women find they have extra energy when they're in the water," notes Dr. Katz.

The Right Footwear

You could swim barefoot. But if you're swimming to shape up, experts recommend the following footwear.

Swim fins. Available at scuba diving shops and sporting goods stores that sell gear for water sports, swim fins help you swim faster—and give your legs a better workout. "Because fins create more resistance against the water for your muscles, you kick faster," says Dr. Katz. "Look for medium-length fins, not the extra-short ones. The length is what's helping you go fast."

Shower sandals. To protect yourself against athlete's foot, a nasty skin infection that is picked up from fungus in and around public pools and showers, you'll want to wear rubber flip-flops, sandals, or water shoes to walk to the pool and also to take a shower, says Dr. Katz. For flip-flops and sandals, the kind sold in discount stores is fine, she says. Water shoes can be found in sporting goods stores that sell water sports gear.

What Else You'll Need

Let's start with the big item.

A pool. Maybe you'll be swimming in a lake or the ocean. But most women who swim regularly are probably doing laps at their local pool or YWCA.

A bathing suit. If you're like a lot of women, the thought of wearing a swimsuit in public makes you cringe. "It's just a matter of getting from the edge of the pool into the water," says Dr. Katz. "Once you're in there, no one can see what you look like."

That said, Dr. Katz advises women who swim for exercise to buy a racing suit designed and produced by sportswear companies. "Shop at a sporting goods store first, rather than a department store," she says. "You're not looking for something to lounge in but rather something that will hold your body in place and keep you streamlined in the water." For exercise swimming, she advises women to stay away from suits with skirts or other added layers of fabric.

Fortunately, the traditional racer-back suit, which is available in almost all sizes, is flattering to almost every figure, since it covers your backside and upper thighs more adequately than fashion swimsuits cut high on the thigh. For large-breasted women, Dr. Katz recommends fitness swimsuits with support. "You can purchase these at specialty fitness stores where swimsuits are geared to accommodate your form."

Finally, Dr. Katz has one other piece of advice for the bathing suit shy: "Swim at a facility that's not too highbrow. More expensive clubs tend to be more looks-oriented, but your local Y caters to every type of body."

Goggles. To minimize levels of harmful bacteria, pool water must contain a certain amount of chlorine and other disinfecting chemicals that can irritate your eyes, so you need goggles. They're a must for swimming laps, says Dr. Katz, because they allow you to see the lane markers along the bottom of the pool. Goggles aren't expensive; pick up a pair at a specialty fitness store where someone

Power Up in the Pool

You'll burn more calories if you go beyond the basic crawl and add other strokes to your repertoire. Try these moves.

Flip onto your back. A major calorie burner (345 calories per half-hour if you weigh 150 pounds), the backstroke is a wonderful complement to the crawl.

Stay on your side. The side stroke doesn't burn the most calories (249 per half-hour), but it is a relaxing way to cool down and work the oblique muscles, located along your torso. Toned obliques mean a toned waistline.

Fly like a butterfly. One of the toughest strokes to master, the butterfly pays off in terms of calories burned (351 per half-hour). If you can master it, you'll feel like a powerhouse in the pool.

Learn the new breaststroke. The breaststroke has been reinvented. It calls for more whip in the kick and a more efficient, faster, narrower arm motion that doesn't strain your muscles as much as the old method. It's also harder than it used to be. But it's still a great way to strengthen your pectoral muscles in your chest (and thus lift your breasts). You'll burn 330 calories per half-hour.

can help you choose the best-fitting ones. (If you're near-sighted, you can even get goggles with an index close to your prescription. They're available for around $30 at specialty stores.) For beginning swimmers, Dr. Katz recommends goggles with good peripheral vision and padding around the rim of the eyepiece. You should feel light suction around the eyes—just enough to keep water out.

A bathing cap. Public pools sometimes require women (and sometimes men) to wear bathing caps. Wearing a cap also helps to protect your hair from chemicals in the pool water, which can dry or discolor your hair. And if your hair is long, a cap keeps it from becoming tangled while you swim. Look for something sleek and simple at a specialty fitness store. A silicone bathing cap is best because it doesn't pull your hair as much as other materials do, explains Dr. Katz.

Soap and a scrubbie. Pool chemicals can dry and irritate your skin if you don't shower with soap and moisturize after you get out of the pool, says Dr. Katz. You can use bar soap and a washcloth, but Dr. Katz says that liquid soap is often easier to carry in your gym bag. Just squirt some on a scrubbie (those balls of nylon that are sold in drugstores), lather up, rinse well, and moisturize when you get out of the shower. Your skin will thank you.

Shampoo and conditioner. Shampoo and condition as soon as possible after each swim, advises Dr. Katz. "Try a shampoo and conditioner formulated to help remove chlorine; these are available at hair salons."

A T-shirt or a robe. If you feel self-conscious about walking from the shower or locker to the pool, Dr. Katz recommends bringing some sort of cover-up to the pool.

Getting Started

"Swimming for exercise is not the same as taking a dip when you're hot and want to cool off after a day in the sun," points out Dr. Katz. "You have to swim at a consistent pace for at least 20 minutes in order to get your heart pumping and your fat burning."

Crawl first. Unless you're proficient in another stroke (breast, back, side, or butterfly), you'll probably want to do the crawl, which is sometimes called freestyle swimming. Before you attempt to learn several strokes, simply work on being able to consistently do a crawl for 10 minutes at a time, says Dr. Katz.

Learn to roll. Sure, swimming looks as if your arms and legs are providing all the power. But the real source of a swimmer's power comes from—surprise—the hips and trunk. "Efficient swimmers are always in a rolling motion," says Dr. Katz. "They're never still in the water." The key is to move from your hips, turning your head to one side to breathe as the opposite arm comes out of the water, then starting to roll toward the other side for your next breath and its matching stroke.

Turn your head and inhale. If you haven't swum laps for a long time, you may feel awkward trying to pace your breaths. When you breathe, turn your whole head along with your body toward one side. Your mouth will lift slightly out of the water for an inhalation. As your body rolls back into a straight line, you'll slowly blow bubbles as you exhale into the water. Continue your body roll to the other side, turning your mouth out of the water on the other side for your next inhalation. Alternating breathing in this way helps to balance your stroke, says Dr. Katz. When you become a proficient swimmer, alternate breathing sides every third pull.

Lead with your head. Your head, not your chin, should lead the way down the lane, says Dr. Katz. You want your body in one streamlined position so that you're looking toward the floor of the pool. Don't worry about hitting the wall—when you see the end of the black line in your lane, start to make your turn and swim back down the lane.

Watch out for other swimmers. If you've joined an aquatic facility, a YWCA, or a gym, chances are you'll be sharing the pool with others, so you have to learn the etiquette of sharing lanes. In some clubs, swimmers do circle-swims, swimming to the right-hand side of the lane and turning counterclockwise at the end of each lap. At other pools, each swimmer has one side of a lane—that is, you stay on one side of the black line that goes down the middle of a lane.

Walking

What could be simpler than putting one foot in front of the other? That's all there is to walking. You don't need fancy equipment, a health club membership, or even good weather. Indoors, you can walk on a treadmill or stride around a mall. Outside, the sky's the limit.

Best of all, walking can give you all the rewards of aerobic exercise, but it puts less stress on your knees, hips, and back. A walking routine can help lower your risk of heart disease, reduce your cholesterol and blood pressure, speed up fat loss, and increase muscle tone, says Rosemary Agostini, M.D., clinical associate professor of orthopedics at the University of Washington and staff physician at the Virginia Mason Sports Medicine Center, both in Seattle.

Body-Shaping Benefits

Here's what you can expect when you walk regularly.

- Your body will burn more calories and more fat all day long because you've revved up your metabolism.

- You'll help tone your abdominals, hips, thighs, and buttocks.
- You'll use all the major muscles—glutes, quads, hamstrings, back, biceps, and triceps.

Psychological Benefits

Walking makes you feel better. If you want proof, just ask the women who take walking classes from nationally known racewalking instructor and coach Bonnie Stein in Redington Shores, Florida. Cynthia Gates Baber, a licensed social worker and psychotherapist at the Scottish Rite Children's Medical Center in Atlanta, conducted a study of 25 women in one of Stein's walking classes. At the start of the 8-week program, Baber discovered that 48 percent of the women showed signs of stress, and almost half had been in therapy for depression. By the end of 8 weeks, only 32 percent of the women showed signs of stress.

The Right Footwear

Priority one for all walkers is good shoes. Here is what Stein recommends that you look for when you shop for shoes.

Flexibility. The shoe should bend where your foot bends—at the ball of your foot, not in the middle of the shoe.

An ample toe box. When you walk, you bend and push off with your toes. There should be a thumb's width from the end of your longest toe to the front end of the shoe, says Stein. If the toe box isn't big enough, your toes will be tingling 20 minutes into your walk.

Light, thin materials. Look for shoes that are lightweight, with a thin heel and a flexible sole. Running and walking shoes with soles that are extremely thick and cushioned are

Customize Your Walking Technique

To maximize the body-shaping benefits of walking, follow these tips from Kate Larsen, a walking instructor and certified group fitness instructor in Minneapolis.

Take short, quick steps instead of long strides. You'll work your glute muscles (in your buttocks) as you log miles.

Practice the heel-toe roll. Push off from your heel, roll through the outside of your foot, then push through your big toe. Think of your big toe as the go button, and push off with propulsion. Keep your other toes relaxed. (This takes practice.)

Squeeze your glutes. Imagine squeezing and lifting your glutes up and back, as if you were holding a $50 bill between them. This will strengthen and tone your glute muscles. Developing the ability to maintain this deep contraction throughout your walk will take a while.

"Zip up" your abs. During your walk, imagine that you're zipping up a tight pair of jeans. Stand tall and pull your abdominal muscles up and in. You can practice this even when you're not walking. This will also strengthen your lower-back muscles.

Pump your arms. Imagine that you're holding the rubber grips of ski poles in your hands. Stand straight, drop your shoulders, squeeze your shoulder blades behind

not good for walking. Also stay away from aerobic, tennis, and basketball shoes, Stein says. Cross-trainers are too stiff and inflexible for walking and don't offer the proper support.

What Else You'll Need

If you venture outdoors on your walks, you'll want to be prepared for any conditions.

you, and push your elbows back with each step. Keep your arm movements smooth and strong, moving past the outside of your hips.

Keep your chest up and shoulders back. Use your walk as an opportunity to practice perfect posture. Imagine that someone dumped ice down your back. That's the feeling you want to have as you hold your chest up and shoulders back.

Hold your head up. Look about 10 feet ahead of you. Imagine that you're wearing a baseball cap with the bill of the visor level to the horizon, so that you have to look up just enough to see the road. This keeps your neck aligned properly.

Smile and have fun. Learning these techniques takes time and concentration. Be patient and enjoy your workouts. Dress comfortably, find a partner, or wear a headset (if you're walking indoors only) and listen to music you love, and if you're walking outdoors, vary your route.

Practice mental fitness. Don't replay the problems of the day while you walk. Try to maintain a state of relaxed awareness by paying attention to your breathing and noticing how your body feels. Visualize and tell yourself you're getting healthier, stronger, and leaner.

Water. Drink 2 cups (16 ounces) of water about 2 hours prior to your workout, then 5 to 10 ounces every 15 to 20 minutes during exercise, says Dr. Agostini. After you're done, drink 16 ounces for each pound of weight lost during the workout.

Sun protection. Wear sunscreen and a floppy, wide-brimmed hat or a baseball cap, sunglasses with 100 percent UV protection, or a visor to shade your eyes and protect your face from sunburn. A visor is best for really hot weather because it doesn't hold the heat in.

Wet-weather gear. There's plenty of rain gear available to make wet-weather walking enjoyable. You can also find wet-weather activewear in mail-order catalogs such as L. L. Bean and Eddie Bauer.

Cold-weather gear. When it's cold outside, you want clothing made with a fabric that pulls the moisture away from your skin. Look for T-shirts, turtlenecks, and other attire made with CoolMax or other synthetic fibers designed for activewear. You can dress in layers, but don't wear cotton next to your skin, because it won't wick away the sweat. Cover your ears with a headband or a hat. Just be aware that even at a cool 35°F or 40°F, a hat may make your head perspire, so a headband is a better choice. When the temperatures dip below freezing, however, wear a hat. When the weather is cool, you may want to wear gloves. When it gets really cold, switch to mittens. Stein likes polar fleece for headbands and mittens because it doesn't trap moisture.

Getting Started

With your walking shoes firmly on your feet, it's time to hit the road. Here are some pointers from Stein.

Take it slow. If you need to lose 50 or more pounds or if you are relatively inactive, don't overdo it at first. Aim for a daily 20-minute walk at a pace that makes your breathing just a bit labored but doesn't leave you out of breath. "At the end of 20 minutes, you'll probably feel great, as though you could do more—but don't," says Stein. "In the first 2 to 3 weeks of walking, don't go more than 20 minutes per session."

Keep going. If you can, walk the entire 20 minutes without stopping. But even if you can walk only 10 minutes at a time, you'll get some benefits. Slow down and rest for a few minutes, then begin again.

Listen to your heart. "The best indicator of whether you're walking briskly enough to gain health benefits is your target heart rate," says Dr. Agostini.

Plan to walk every day. "Even on days when you don't feel like doing it, just get out and walk a few blocks," says Stein. You'd be surprised at how, once you get going, those few blocks can turn into a mile or more.

If you're an indoor walker, consider buying a treadmill. Stein recommends a motorized version. Set it at a speed that lets you walk comfortably without holding on. When you feel balanced and are used to it, you can increase the speed. Walk on a treadmill for the same amount of time you would if you were walking outside.

Index